Natural Products Chemistry Practical Manual

(For Science and Pharmacy Courses)

W0081029

Natural Products Chemistry Practical Manual

(For Science and Pharmacy Courses)

Dr. Anees A. Siddiqui
Department of Pharmaceutical Chemistry
Faculty of Pharmacy
Jamia Hamdard, Hamdard Nagar
New Delhi-110062

Seemi Siddiqui
SCG College of Pharmacy
Ahera (Baghpat)

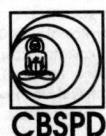

CBSPD

CBS Publishers & Distributors Pvt Ltd

New Delhi • Bengaluru • Chennai • Kochi • Kolkata • Lucknow • Mumbai
Hyderabad • Jharkhand • Nagpur • Patna • Pune • Uttarakhand

Natural Products Chemistry
Practical Manual

(For Science and Pharmacy Courses)

ISBN-13: 978-81-239-1621-7

Copyright © Publisher

First Edition: 2008

Reprint: 2012, 2017, 2019, **2024**

All rights reserved. No part of this book may be reproduced or transmitted in any form or by any means, electronic or mechanical, including photocopying, recording or any information storage and retrieval system without permission, in writing from the author and publisher.

Published by **Satish Kumar Jain** and produced by **Varun Jain** for
CBS Publishers & Distributors Pvt Ltd
4819/XI Prahlad Street, 24 Ansari Road, Daryaganj, New Delhi 110 002, India
Ph: 011-23289259, 23266861   Website: www.cbspd.com
                                           e-mail: delhi@cbspd.com

Corporate Office: 204 FIE, Industrial Area, Patparganj, Delhi 110 092, India
Ph: 011-4934 4934   Fax: 011-4934 4935   e-mail: publishing@cbspd.com;
                                                   publicity@cbspd.com

Branches

- **Bengaluru:** Seema House 2975, 17th Cross, KR Road, Banasankari 2nd Stage, Bengaluru 560 070, Karnataka, India
  Ph: +91-80-26771678/79   Fax: +91-80-26771680   e-mail: bangalore@cbspd.com
- **Chennai:** 7, Subbaraya Street, Shenoy Nagar, Chennai 600 030, Tamil Nadu, India
  Ph: +91-44-26680620, 26681266   Fax: +91-44-42032115   e-mail: chennai@cbspd.com
- **Kochi:** 42/1325, 1326, Power House Road, Opp KSEB, Power House, Ernakulum Kochi 682 018, Kerala, India
  Ph: +91-484-4059061-65,67   Fax: +91-484-4059065   e-mail: kochi@cbspd.com
- **Kolkata:** 147, Hind Ceramics Compound, 1st Floor, Nilgunj Road, Belghoria, Kolkata-700056, West Bengal, India
  Ph: +033-25633055, 033-25633056   e-mail: kolkata@cbspd.com
- **Lucknow:** Basement, Khushnuma Complex, 7 Meerabai Marg (Behind Jawahar Bhawan), Lucknow-226001, UP, India
  Ph: +91-522-4000032   e-mail: tiwari.lucknow@cbspd.com
- **Mumbai:** PWD Shed, Gala no 25/26, Ramchandra Bhatt Marg, Next to JJ Hospital Gate no. 2, Opp. Union Bank of India Noorbaug, Mumbai-400009, Maharashtra, India
  Ph: 022-66661880/89   e-mail: mumbai@cbspd.com

Representatives

- Hyderabad   0-9885175004
- Patna   0-9334159340
- Jharkhand   0-9811541605
- Pune   0-9664372571
- Nagpur   0-8692091830
- Uttarakhand   0-9716462459

Printed at SRK Graphics, Delhi (India)

Preface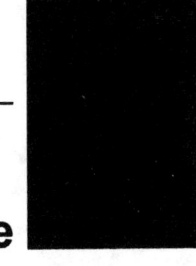

The lack of material for directed laboratory investigations in the area of Phytochemistry or Chemistry of Natural Products has prompted the compiling of this mannul. The Phytochemistry or Chemistry of Natural Products is a part of curriculum in the field of Science and Pharmacy whether it is a under graduate course or PG cource. While student interest and enrolment in these field, continue to increase, a search of the literature indicates relatively little material available in laboratory experiments and almost none in Pharmaceutical area. This laboratory manual is designed to meet the needs in both disciplines and as such with hopefully be considered by faculty in Pharmacy or Science programs in undergraduate or PG courses.

16 major subjects are presented and supported by 101 experiments which is, admittedly far in excess of what could be covered in an academic year in pharmacy or Science courses. But, it is the breadth and diversity of categories that is deliberately designed to allow faculty in various specilities to pick and choose the ones, most relevant to their teaching field. Thus, the subject of Pharmaceutical Chemistry will cover the experiments relating to carbohydrates, lipids , proteins, steroids, and vitamins whereas Chemistry of Natural products or Phytochemistry might choose activities relating to tannins, gums, resins, balsams, glycosides, volatile oils among others.

It is author's hope that the experiments included in this manual will fulfil the need of both programs, Science and Pharmacy.

Comments on the material are always welcome which will be required for the improvisation in the next edition.

Contents

Carbohydrates

Contents

Introduction to Carbohydrates

Carbohydrates are either polyhydroxy aldehydes or ketoses or substances that give these compounds upon hydrolysis. Hence, these are also known as aldoses and ketoses. The most common carbohydrate used by body in energy metabolism is glucose- hexose monosaccharide:

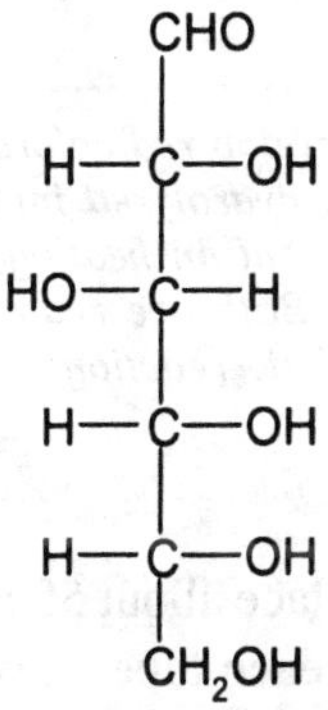

Straight chain formula 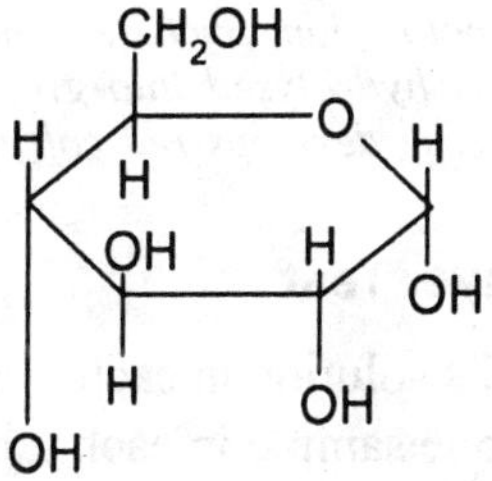   Haworth formulae

Reducing and non reducing Sugars

Alkaline copper solution readily oxidizes many mono- and disaccharides (which contain free carbonyl functional group). During oxidation of sugar molecule, the cupric ion(Cu^{2+}) is reduced into cuprous ion(Cu^{1+}) compound, which can be identified by the color change from deep blue to a red or reddish brown. The sugars that are oxidized by alkaline solution are called reducing sugars.

$$(C_5H_{11}O_5)-CHO + 2Cu^{2+} + 4OH^- \longrightarrow (C_5H_{11}O_5)-CHO + Cu_2O + 2H_2O$$

Glucose   Cuprous oxide
                                                                          (red precipitate)

3

The best known solution/reagent for these tests are:-

- Fehling's solution(an alkaline NaOH, $CuSO_4$ solution with potassium sodium tartrate)
- Benedict's solution(an alkaline Na_2CO_3-$CuSO_4$ in presence of sodium citrate)
- Barfoed's solution(copper acetate in 0.15N acetic acid solution).

The following test is used to differentiate between reducing and non reducing sugars. Take 10ml of Benedict' solution or equal volume of Fehling solution I and II in each of six test tube. Add about 50mg of glucose to the first, fructose to the second, starch to the third, sucrose to the fourth, lactose to the fifth and in the sixth starch with 10 ml of saliva. Shake well and allow the tubes to stand for 15 minutes. Then, heat the each tube gently on water bath for 10-15 minutes. Record the result in the table:

Sugar	Color reaction	Reducing(Check)
1. Glucose	–	–
2. Fructose	–	–
3. Starch	–	–
4. Lactose	–	–
5. Sucrose	–	–
6. Starch with saliva	–	–

Note. Glucose, fructose, etc are reducing sugars so develop red coloration. Starch is non reducing sugar but in presence of saliva it is hydrolysed into glucose so shows red coloration. Sucrose is non reducing sugar but on heating in presence of HCl, it is hydrolysed into glucose and fructose. Both are reducing sugars. Hence, sucrose develops red colration due to hydrolytic reaction.

Barfoed's Qualitative Test

Place 10ml of Barfoed's solution in each of four test tubes. Place about 50 mg of glucose, fructose, maltose and sucrose, one sample in each tube. Warm gently each tube on water bath and carefully time each reaction

Barfoed's test is similar to Benedict's test, but determines if a carbohydrate is a monosaccharide or a disaccharide. Barfoed's reagent reacts with monosaccharides to produce cuprous oxide at a faster rate than disaccharides do:

$$RCHO + 2Cu^{2+} + 2H_2O \longrightarrow RCOOH + Cu_2O + 4H^+$$

Some Color Tests of Carbohydrates

Due to their diverse molecular structures, the carbohydrates form numerous color complexes with specific reagents. This forms the basis of their identification, sometimes not specifically, but at least as to class as, for example, mono- or disaccharides and hexose or pentose.

Molisch Test

In each of four test tubes, place 1 ml of dilute solution of glucose, xylose and furfural. Add 2 drops of fresh 5% alpha naphthol solution in alcohol directly to each substance. Mix each well, the add 2ml of concentrated H_2SO_4 to flow down the side of each tube to form a lower layer of acid. The appearance of red rings at the interface of two liquid indicates the presence of carbohydrates.

Result :

Glucose ———————

Xylose ———————

Starch ———————

Furfural ———————

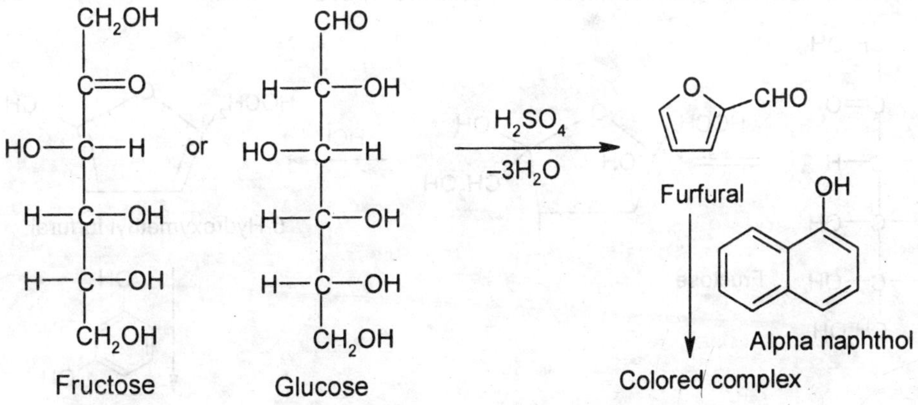

Fructose   Glucose   Furfural   Alpha naphthol   Colored complex

In this test, concentrated H_2SO_4 forms furfurals due to its dehydrating action on carbohydrates. *The furfurals condense with alpha naphthol to form colored products.*

A negative result by this reaction is a good evidence of the absence of carbohydrates, but a positive test is simply an indicator of the probable presence of carbohydrates. Among the substances that give the test are various furfurals, glucuronic acid, erythrose, and glyceraldehydes. The reaction can be made more valuable by examining the absorption spectra of the alcoholic solution of colored condensation products.

Seliwanoff test

This is an indicative test for hexoses but heto-hexoses, keto-trioses, keto-tetroses, d-oxygluconic acid & formose also react positively. Prepare fresh Seliwanoff by adding 3.5 ml of 0.5% fresh resorcinol to 12ml of concentrated HCl and dilute to 35 ml with distilled water.

Place 5ml of glucose, galactose, levulose, xylose and furfural respectively into 5 different test tubes. Add 5ml of above freshly prepared Seliwanoff reagent to each tube. Mix well and warm gently on boiling water bath for 15 minutes. Observe the color change.

Results :

Glucose   ——————
Galactose   ——————
Levulose   ——————
Xylose   ——————
Furfural   ——————

Seilwanoff's Test is a test for ketoses. In this test, concentrated HCl is used. Ketoses usually dehydrate at a faster rate than do aldoses, allowing for the discrimination of the two. The limit of detection is 20 mg/mL. A positive test is the formation of orange to red color within 5 minutes without the formation of a precipitate. Sucrose also tests positive with this test. An apricot color is not a positive test. It is interesting to note that glucose gives no color even after 10 minutes. The color developed here is due to the formation of 4-hydroxy methyl furfural and reaction of this with resorcinol in the presence of HCl solution.

Fructose

5-Hydroxymethyl furfural

Colored complex

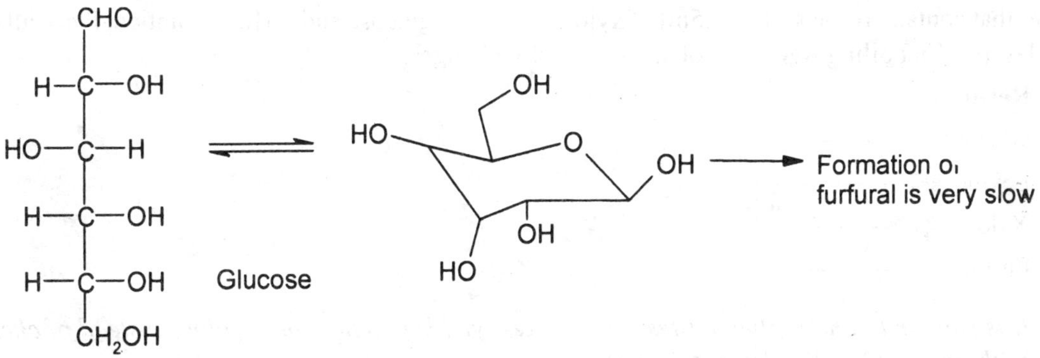

Glucose

Tollen's Phloroglucinol Test

Prepare a fresh reagent by mixing 10ml of concentrated HCl with 2ml of the phloroglucinol solution and dilute to 20ml with water. Measure of 5ml portion of this solution and add, respectively, to tubes containing 0.5ml of xylose, levulose, glucose and furfural solution. Place all but the last tube in the boiling water and note color changes over 15 minutes.

Result:

Glucose   ——————

Levulose   ——————

Xylose   ——————

Furfural   ——————

This reaction is positive for pentoses, but not a specific indication of them since hexoses and glucuronic acid also react. If the cherry red color develops very promptly, and if this is soluble in amyl alcohol, then it can be considered a fairly reliable test for pentoses and glucuronic acid. The colored compounds formed are condensation products of various intermediate and final decomposition products from carbohydrates with the phenolic compound phloroglucinol(1,3,5-trihydroxy benzene).

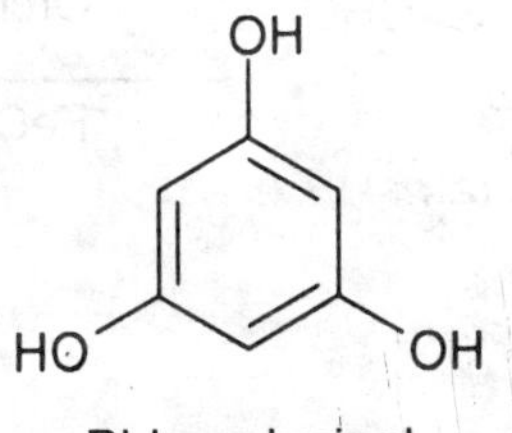

Phloroglucinol

Tollen's Orcinol Test

Prepare a fresh reagent by mixing 10ml of concentrated HCl with 2ml of a 6% aqueous solution of orcinol and dilute it to 20 ml with water. Now measure off 5ml portion of the orcinol reagent into test tubes that contain, respectively, 0.5ml of xylose, levulose, glucose and furfural solution. Place all but the last tube in boiling water and observe the color changes.

Result :

Glucose ⎯⎯⎯⎯⎯

Levulose ⎯⎯⎯⎯⎯

Xylose ⎯⎯⎯⎯⎯

Furfural ⎯⎯⎯⎯⎯

It is similar to phloroglucinol test but this test yields greenish-blue colors instead of cherry red with orcinol(3,5 dihydroxy toluene).

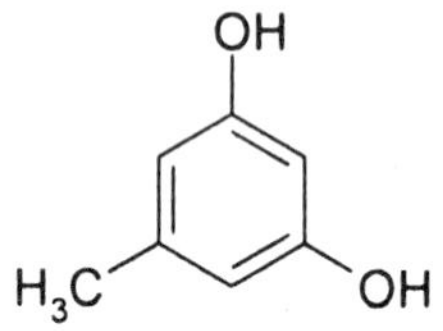

Orcinol

Bials test

Take two ml of a sample solution in a test tube. Add two ml of Bial's reagent (a solution of orcinol, HCl and ferric chloride) is added. Heat the solution gently in a Bunsen Burner or hot water bath. If the color is not obvious, more water can be added to the tube.

It is a test for pentoses. In the presence of concentrated HCl, the furfural that is produced as in Salwanoffs test) generates a blue-green color in the presence of orcinol and ferric ions.

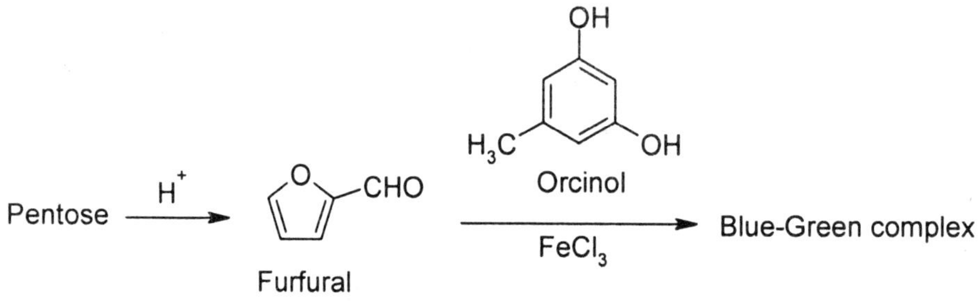

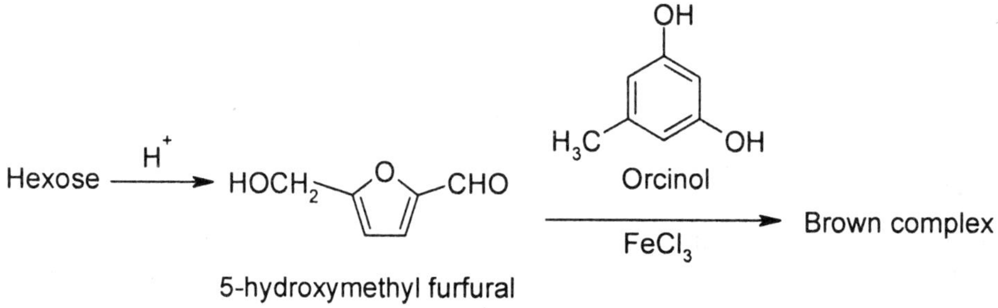

Thus a positive test is the formation of a bluish green color within 5 minutes, again without the formation of a precipitate. Note that hexoses generally react to form green, red, or brown products. Di- and polysaccharides give the same results but at a much slower rate.

Iodine Test

1. Number three clean test tubes: 1, 2, & 3 and add a carbohydrate solution to each:
   - Tube 1–20 drops of glucose (monosaccharide) solution
   - Tube 2–20 drops of sucrose (disaccharide) solution
   - Tube 3–20 drops of starch (polysaccharide) solution
2. Add 4 drops of iodine solution to each tube.
3. Mix the contents of each tube by gently swirling.
4. Record **in Data table** the color of the solutions in the three tubes in the column marked "Iodine color".

Color change may or may not occur when iodine solution is added to a carbohydrate. A change from its original rustcolor to a deep blue-black occurs if a polysaccharide is present. The original color of the iodine remains in a disaccharide or monosaccharide sugar is present.

Red Tetrazolium Test

Several tests have been developed over the years to determine whether a sugar is reducing or not. Fehling's and Benedict's tests are classic ones that rely on copper ions. Tollen's test, which relies on silver ions, has also been used. Red Tetrazolium Test"is highly sensitive, not too hazardous, and the reagent is very easy to prepare.

Into test tube, place two (Pasteur pipet) drops of your unknown carbohydrate solution. Add 1 mL of 0.5% aqueous red tetrazolium reagent and 1 drop of 3M NaOH. Mix and place the test tubes in a beaker of hot water. Record the time it takes for each tube to develop an intense red color.

The reagent (2,3,5-triphenyl-2H-tetrazolium chloride) is colorless and water-soluble and undergoes the following reaction:

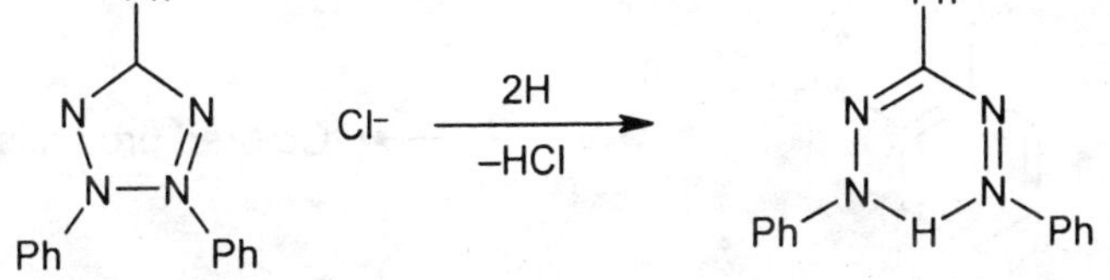

"Red tetrazolium" (colorless)   Red tetrazolium-diformazan-red

Red tetrazolium is easily reduced in hot basic solution, and converted into an insoluble red product. The test is very sensitive so be sure to work with very clean test tubes.

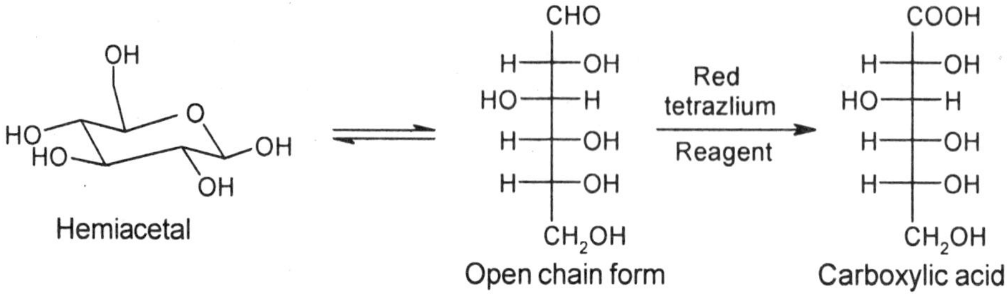

Hemiacetal ⇌ Open chain form → Carboxylic acid

Hydrolysis Test for Glucose

Disaccharides and polysaccharides can be hydrolyzed in acidic solution into their component monosaccharides, and then submitted to chemical tests like Benedict's test. In this experiment, several disaccharides and a sample of starch will be hydrolyzed, and tested for the presence of glucose. The glucose test will be carried out using a commercially available product called *Test-Tape or Test strip. Available at most drug stores, the tape contains the enzymes glucose oxidase and peroxidase, as well as ortho-toluidine. The glucose oxidase oxidizes glucose to gluconic acid and hydrogen peroxide. Once formed, the hydrogen peroxide reacts with peroxidase to produce oxygen, which oxidizes the ortho-toluidine to give green-colored products.*

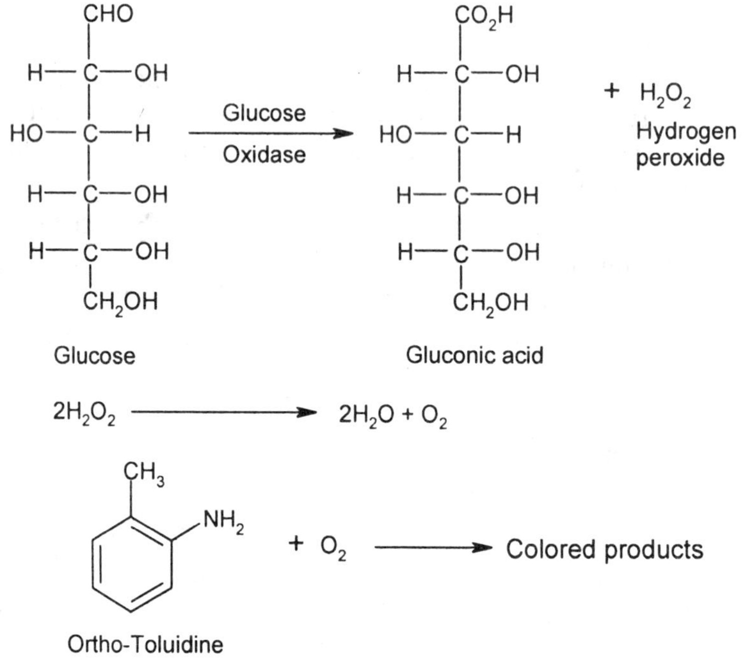

Glucose → Gluconic acid + H_2O_2 (Hydrogen peroxide)

$$2H_2O_2 \longrightarrow 2H_2O + O_2$$

Ortho-Toluidine + O_2 ⟶ Colored products

Place 5 mL of the following 1% carbohydrate solutions in separate, labelled test tubes: sucrose, lactose, maltose, and starch. Add 3 drops of concentrated hydrochloric acid to each of the tubes, and heat them in a boiling water bath (400 mL beaker) for 10 minutes. Cool the tubes in an ice bath.

Carefully neutralize each of the four solutions with 10% sodium hydroxide, using litmus or pH paper. **The pH MUST be neutral or very slightly alkaline in order for the Tes-Tape to work.** If necessary, make final pH adjustments with 0.1M HCl and/or 0.1M NaOH solutions. Test each solution with Tes-Tape (by placing a drop on the tape and recording the color change - use plain distilled water as a control) and if time permits, with Benedict's reagent. Record the results and compare them with those obtained earlier with the Benedict's tests on the unhydrolysed carbohydrates.

Production of Ethanol from Sucrose

The ethyl alcohol is commercially obtained by fermentation process of carbohydrate, sucrose. It is a disaccharide, $C_{12}H_{22}O_{11}$; has one glucose molecule combined with fructose. The enzyme, zymase converts the sugar to ethyl alcohol and carbon dioxide. For experimental production of ethyl alcohol, there is need of Pasteur's salts. This consists of 2.0 gm of potassium phosphate, 0.20gm magnesium sulphate, 0.20 gm of calcium phosphate and 10 gm of ammonium tartrate dissolved in 860 ml of water.

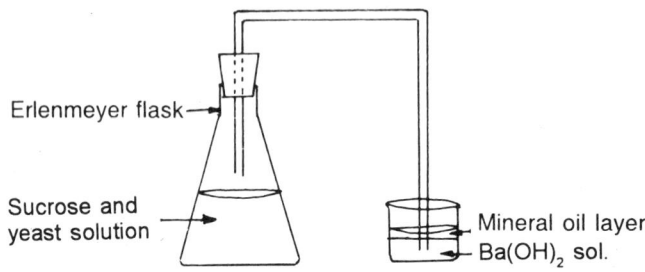

Fig 3.1. Production of ethanol

Place 40 gm of sucrose in a 500 ml of Erlenmeyer flask. Add 350ml of water, 35 ml of Pasteur's salts and 15 gm of beaker's yeast. Shake vigorously and fit the flask with one-hole rubber stopper with a glass tube leading to a beaker containing a solution of barium hydroxide. Protect the barium hydroxide from air by adding some mineral oil to form a layer over it. A precipitate of barium carbonate will eventually form indicating the evolution of carbon dioxide.

$$Ba(OH)_2 + CO_2 \longrightarrow BaCO_3 + H_2O$$

Allow the mixture to stand 1 week before proceeding. After this period of time, carefully remove the rubber stopper and siphon off the liquid from the flask, being careful not to disturb the sediment. Add 46 gm of anhydrous potassium carbonate for each 100ml of solution, which, in effect, saturates the solution. Transfer to a distillation apparatus and slowly heat until a temperature of 78°C is reached. At this point discard any distillate collected and begin to collect the ethyl alcohol. Do not heat beyond 88°C. Discard the residue in the flask and measure the volume of ethyl alcohol collected.

Calculate the percentage yield of ethyl alcohol based on an average yield of 85% water and 15% alcohol.

It may be noted here that when disaccharide is used in fermentation, the enzyme in yeast first converts into a mixture of invert sugar(glucose and fructose), which then undergoes fermentation according to the equation:

$$C_{12}H_{22}O_{11} \longrightarrow 2C_2H_5OH + 2CO_2$$

$$\frac{\text{Actual yield}}{\text{Theoretical yield}} \times 100 = \text{.......} \% \text{ yield}$$

Isolation of Lactose from Milk

Lactose, which is the popular name for milk sugar, can be isolated from milk by a fairly simple laboratory procedure. It is a disaccharide with the structural formula of:

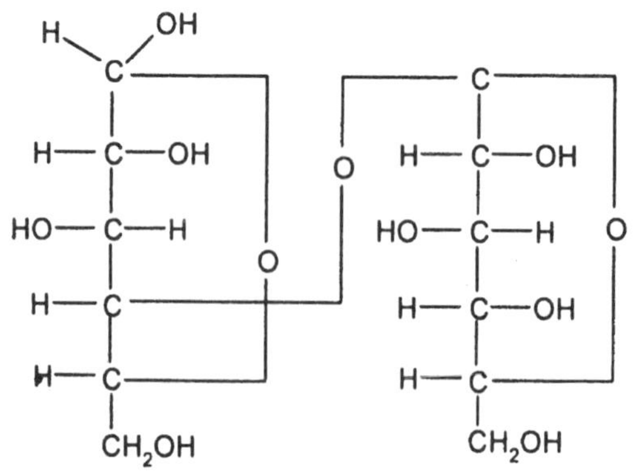

Lactose

(i) Place 200 ml of skimmed (nonfat) milk in a 600 ml beaker and warm it to 40°C; then add dropwise some 10% acetic acid until there is a significant precipitate of casein. Do not add excess acid as it may hydrolyse the disaccharide, lactose to the monosaccharide glucose and galactose. Stir the casein until it forms a large amorphous mass and remove it from the mixture.

(ii) The clear solution now consists the lactose which we want to isolate. Add 5 gm $CaCO_3$ to the clear solution. Heat this mixture to a gentle boil for about 10 minutes. This should result in the nearly complete precipitation of the albumin.

(iii) Filter the hot mixture by vacuum to remove the precipitated albumins plus remaining $CaCO_3$ and concentrate the filtrate in a 600 ml beaker, using a water bath, to about 30ml. Do not boil too vigorously otherwise excessive foaming may occur. Some marble chips may be added in mixture to prevent bumping.

(iv) Now add 175 ml of 95% ethanol and 2gm of decolorizing charcoal to the hot solution. After, it has been mixed well, filter the warm solution by vacuum through a layer of wet filter(diatomaceous earth). Make sure the filtrate is clear.

(v) Transfer the filtrate to a flask and allow it to stand for several days. This provides time for the lactose to crystallize and vacuum filter them. Wash the product with 10ml of 25% ehyl alcohol.

(vi) Weigh the product after it is thoroughly dry.

Results: ————— gm

(vii) Using the density of skimmed milk 1.03 gm/ml, calculate the percentage yield of lactose.

Benedict's test for identification of lactose

To a solution of 1% lactose in distilled water, add 5ml Benedict's solution and heat gently on a boiling water bath for 5 minutes and observe the color change.

Determination of Total Lactose in Milk and Milk Powders (Gravimetric method)

1. Principle

The method is based on reduction of a cupric salt complex to Cu_2O under specified conditions by lactose. The amount of Cu_2O precipitated is proportional to the lactose content.

2. Scope

The method is used on all milk and whey powders.

3. Reagents

1. Fehling I.
   Copper(II)sulphate solution.
   Dissolve 34.639 gm $CuSO_4$, $5H_2O$ in deionized water.
   Dilute to 500.0 ml in a volumetric flask, and filter through a paper filter.
   Store in a 500 ml brown glass bottle.

2. Fehling II.
   Alkaline tartrate solution.
   Dissolve 173.0 ± 0.1 gm $C_4H_4Na_2O_6$, H_2O and 50.0 ± 0.1 g NaOH pellets in deionized water and dilute to 500 ml in a volumetric flask. Allow to stand for 2 days, before filtering through a paper filter.
   Store in a 500 ml brown glass bottle.

3. Potassium hydroxide solution.
   Dissolve 15.567 gm KOH in deionized water. Dilute to 500.0 ml in a volumetric flask.

Procedure

1. Weigh out according to type of powder ± 0.05 gm:
   Milk powder   1.60 gm

Skim milk   2.00 gm
Whole milk   2.80 gm

2. Dissolve the powder in approx. 200 ml 60°C deionized water in a 500 ml volumetric flask. Invert the solution until all powder is dissolved, and cool to 20°C. Filter the solution (F4)

3. Add 10 ml of Fehling I solution and 7.5 ml (measuring pipette) KOH solution (the solution must still be acidic, check with litmus (pH) paper), and dilute to 500.0 ml.

4. Mix carefully and filter through a dry filter (F4).

5. Pipette 25.0 ml of Fehling I solution and 25.0 ml of Fehling II solution into a 400 ml beaker.

6. Add 25 ml of the filtrate (F4) and 25 ml of deionized water.

7. Cover the beaker with a watch glass and heat it over a Bunsen burner or a hot plate.
   The heat must be regulated so boiling begins after 4 minutes.
   Continue boiling for exactly 2 minutes.
   It is important that these regulations are strictly maintained.
   For this purpose it is recommended to make a preliminary test, using 50 ml deionized water and 50 ml reagent.

8. Filter the solution immediately through a dried and weighed glass filter crucible by means of suction.

9. Transfer the precipitated Cu_2O quantitatively to the glass filter crucible, and wash it carefully, first with 60°C deionized water, then with 10 ml alcohol and finally with 10 ml of ether.

10. Dry the precipitate in an oven at 100°C for 30 minutes, cool in a desiccator and weigh.

11. Carry out a blank test according to step 5 to 10 using deionized water instead of reducing sugar filtrate. If the weight of the Cu_2O obtained in the blank is more than 0.5 mg, correct the results of reducing sugar determination accordingly.

7. Result

Use the **Hammond Table** to express the weight of lactose equivalent to the weight of Cu_2O.

$$\% \text{ lactose in powder} = \frac{A \times 500 \times 100}{W \times ml \times 1000}$$

A = mg lactose equivalent to the weight of Cu_2O as found in the table.
W = weight of milk powder
ml = ml filtrate taken with pipette

Hammond table for calculating lactose values expressed in mg

Cu_2O	Lactose, H_2O	Cu_2O	Lactose, H_2O
20	13.6	76	51.7
30	20.2	77	52.4
40	27.2	78	53.0

(Contd.)

Cu_2O	Lactose, H_2O	Cu_2O	Lactose, H_2O
50	34.0	79	53.7
51	34.7	80	54.4
52	35.4	81	55.1
53	36.0	82	55.8
54	36.7	83	56.4
55	37.4	84	57.1
56	38.1	85	57.8
57	38.8	86	58.5
58	39.4	87	59.2
59	40.1	88	59.8
60	40.8	89	60.5
61	41.5	90	61.2
62	42.2	91	61.9
63	42.9	92	62.6
64	43.5	93	63.2
65	44.2	94	63.9
66	44.9	95	64.6
67	45.6	96	65.3
68	46.2	97	66.0
69	46.9	98	66.6
70	47.6	99	67.3
71	48.3	100	68.0
72	49.0	150	102.3
73	49.6	200	136.6
74	50.3	250	171.1
75	51.0	300	205.7

Isolation of Mucic acid from Galactose

When a strong HNO_3 solution is heated with an aldose hexose, it oxidizes to the corresponding dicarboxylic acid. Most of the aldoses yield the soluble dicarboxylic acid but galactose or lactose yields mucic acid, which is sparingly soluble in water. Nitric acid oxidizes the terminal groups of aldoses but leave the secondary hydroxyl group unchanged.

$$C_6H_{12}O_6 + 6HNO_3 \longrightarrow HCOO(CHOH)_4COOH + 4H_2O + 6NO_2$$
$$\text{Mucic acid}$$

It forms a crystalline powder which melts at 213°C. It is insoluble in alcohol, and nearly insoluble in cold water. When heated with pyridine to 140°C, it is converted into allommic acid. When digested with fuming hydrochloric acid for some time, it is converted into a furfural dicarboxylic acid while on heating with barium sulphide, it is transformed into a thiophene carboxylic acid. The ammonium salt yields on dry distillation carbon dioxide, ammonia, pyrrol and other substances. The acid when fused with caustic alkalis yields oxalic acid.

With potassium bisulphite, mucic acid forms **3-hydroxy-2-pyrone** by dehydration and decarboxylation.

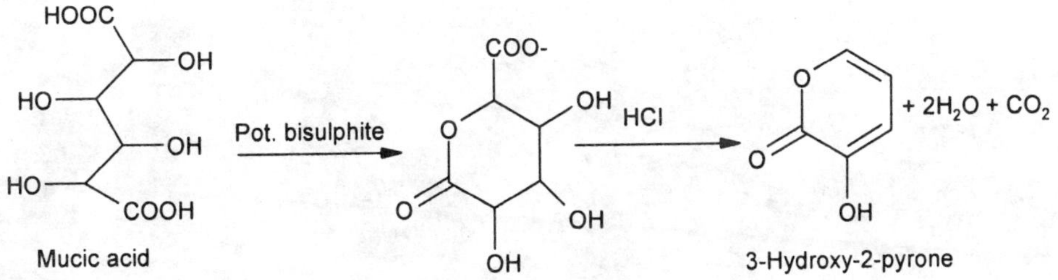

Mucic acid → Pot. bisulphite → HCl → 3-Hydroxy-2-pyrone $+ 2H_2O + CO_2$

Isolation procedure

(i) To 25 ml of 0.1M lactose or galactose solution in a 100 ml beaker, add 10ml of distilled water and 15 ml HNO_3.

(ii) Mix well and heat on a steam bath until concentrated to about one third the original volume. Then add 10ml of distilled water and mix well. Set aside in a cool place until the next day.

(iii) Filter the mucic acid crystals, dry and weigh the product.

(iv) Calculate the percentage yield by comparing the actual yield based on the formula stochiometry.

$$\frac{\text{Actual yield}}{\text{Theoretical yield}} \times 100 = \text{........} \% \text{ yield}$$

The Chemistry and Isolation of Pectin

Pectin is classified as a soluble fiber. It is found in most of the plants, but is most concentrated in citrus fruits (oranges, lemons, grapefruits) and apples. Pectin is obtained by the aqueous extraction of citrus peels and apple pulp under mild acidic conditions. Pectin obtained from citrus peels, is referred to as citrus pectin.

Pectin is widely used in the food industry as a gelling agent to impart a gelled texture to foods, mainly fruit-based foods such as jams and jellies. It also has pharmaceutical applications. Pectin is used in combination with the clay kaolin (hydrated aluminum silicate) for the management of diarrhea. It is used as a component in the adhesive part of ostomy rings. Pectin is also marketed as a nutritional supplement for the management of elevated cholesterol.

Chemically, pectin is a linear polysaccharide containing from about 300 to 1,000 monosaccharide units. D-Galacturonic acid is the principal monosaccharide unit of pectin. Some neutral sugars are also present in the substance. The D-galacturonic acid residues are linked together by alpha-1, 4 glycosidic linkages. The molecular weight of pectin ranges from 50,000 to 150,000 daltons. The galacturonic acid residues in pectin may be esterified with methyl groups. There are different types of pectin. Pectin in which more than 50% of the galacturonic acid residues are esterified is called high methoxyl or HM pectin. Pectin in which less than 50% of the galacturonic acid residues are esterified is called low methoxy or LM pectin. Pectin is a nondigestible polysaccharide. So-called

Structure of Pectin

modified citrus pectin is pectin that has been hydrolyzed and otherwise modified to make it more digestible and absorbable.

Pectin, is available as white to light brown powder. It was first isolated and described in 1825 by Henri Braconnot.

Experimental procedure

Follow the below given flow chart for its isolation :

Flow Chart for Isolation of Pectin

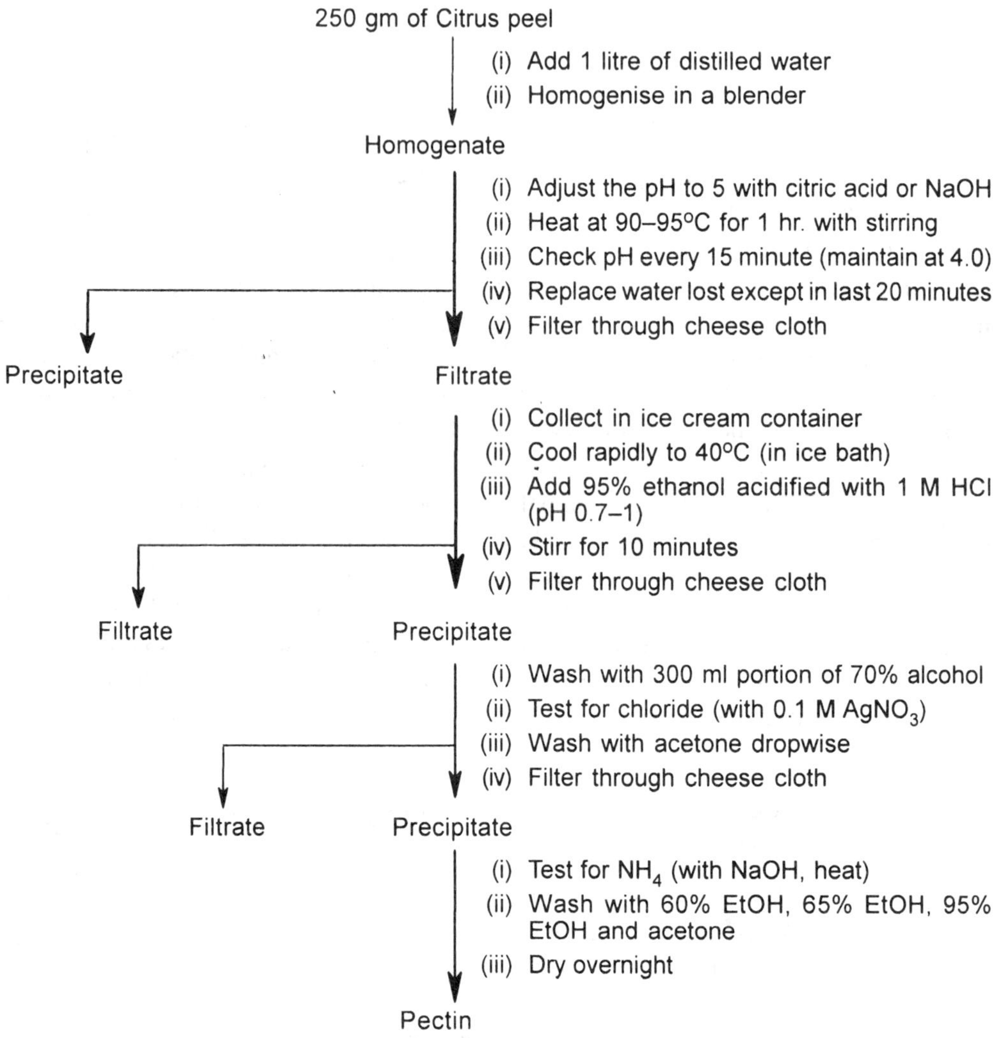

250 gm of Citrus peel

    (i) Add 1 litre of distilled water
    (ii) Homogenise in a blender

Homogenate

    (i) Adjust the pH to 5 with citric acid or NaOH
    (ii) Heat at 90–95°C for 1 hr. with stirring
    (iii) Check pH every 15 minute (maintain at 4.0)
    (iv) Replace water lost except in last 20 minutes
    (v) Filter through cheese cloth

Precipitate   Filtrate

    (i) Collect in ice cream container
    (ii) Cool rapidly to 40°C (in ice bath)
    (iii) Add 95% ethanol acidified with 1 M HCl (pH 0.7–1)
    (iv) Stirr for 10 minutes
    (v) Filter through cheese cloth

Filtrate   Precipitate

    (i) Wash with 300 ml portion of 70% alcohol
    (ii) Test for chloride (with 0.1 M $AgNO_3$)
    (iii) Wash with acetone dropwise
    (iv) Filter through cheese cloth

Filtrate   Precipitate

    (i) Test for NH_4 (with NaOH, heat)
    (ii) Wash with 60% EtOH, 65% EtOH, 95% EtOH and acetone
    (iii) Dry overnight

Pectin

Result:————gm

Calculate the pectin % in the rind.

Assay of Pectins for Methoxyl Groups

Transfer 5 gm of the pectin to a 500 ml beaker and agitate with a magnetic stirrer for 10 minutes with 5ml of dilute HCl and 100 ml of ethyl alcohol (60%). Transfer to a fritted glass filter tube and wash with six 15 ml portion of HCl-60% ethyl alcohol to free the mixture of chlorides. Dry for 1hour in a drying oven at 105°C, cool and weigh. Now transfer exactly one-tenth of the total net weight of the dried sample to a 250 ml Erlenmeyer flask and moisten the sample with 2 ml alcohol. Add 100 ml of recently boiled and cooled H_2O, stopper and swirl occasionally until the pectin is completely dissolved. Add 5 drops phenolphthalein and titrate with 0.5N NaOH and record results as the initial titre. Add 20 ml of 0.5 N NaOH again, stopper and swirl. Let stand for 15 minutes. Add exactly 20 ml of 0.5N HCl and shake until the pink colors disappears After adding 3 drops of phenolphthalein titrate with 0.5N NaOH to a persistent faint pink color. Each ml of the 0.5N NaOH is the saponification titre and equivalent to 15.52 mg of methoxy(–OCH3) on an undried basis.

$$\text{Result: } \text{———ml (NaOH)} \times 15.52 = \text{———mg (–OCH}_3)$$

Assay for Galacturonic Acid

Each ml of the 0.5N NaOH used in the total titration used in the total titration(initial plus saponification) is the equivalent of 97.07 mg of galacturonic acid($C_5H_5O_5COOH$) on an undried basis

Results

Initial titre ——————— ml NaOH

Saponification titre ——————— ml NaOH

Total = ——————— ml NaOH

X 97.07 = ——————— mg galacturonic acid

Determination of Gluten in Semolina(suji)

Wet gluten in durum wheat is a plastic-elastic substance, made of gliadin and glutenin, which is obtained by means of the method specified below. The quality of gluten in wheat is determined by centrifuging a gluten sample taken from a wheat dough against a sieve. Upon completion of the centrifugation process, it is determined how large a proportion of the sample has remained in the sieve, without penetrating there through. The magnitude of this proportion is used as a measurement of the gluten quality.

Principle

Gluten separated from durum whole meals or semolina by Glutomatic method (is centrifuged to force wet gluten through a specially constructed sieve under standardized conditions). The percentage of wet gluten remaining on the sieve after centrifugation is defined as the Gluten Index. If the gluten is very weak all of the gluten may pass through the sieve, the Gluten Index is 0. When nothing passes through the sieve, the Index is 100.

Procedure

Weigh 25 gm of sample into a dish and add about 15ml of water to it and make it into dough taking care that all the material is taken into dough. Keep the dough gently in a beaker filled with the water and let it stand for 1 hr. Remove the dough and place it in a piece of bolting silk cloth with an aperture of 0.16 mm (No.10) and wash it with a gentle stream of water till water passing through the silk does not give a blue color with a drop of iodine solution. Spread the silk tight on a porcelain plate to facilitate scrapping. Collect the residue to form a ball, squeeze in palms to remove water, transfer to a watch glass or Petri dish and keep it in the oven at 105ºC $\pm$ for drying. When partially dried, remove and cut into several pieces with a scissor and again keep in the oven to dry. Cool in desicator and weigh. Return it to the oven again for half hour, cool and weigh to ensure constant weight.

$$\text{Gluten on dry weight basis} = \frac{\text{Weight of dry gluten} \times 100 \times 100}{25 \times (100 - \text{moisture content})}$$

Determination of moisture content

Weigh accurately about 5 gm in a previously dried and tared dish and place the dish with its lid underneath in the ove maintained at 130-133°C for 2 hrs. The time should be reckoned from the moment the oven attains 130°C after the dishes have been placed. Remove the dish after 2 hrs, cool in the desicator and weigh.

$$\text{Moisture content} = \frac{W_1 - W_2}{Wt - W} \times 100$$

W1 = Wt in gm of the dish with material before drying.

W2 = Wt in gm of the dish with material after drying.

W = Wt in gm of the empty dish.

9

Isolation of Glycogen from Liver Tissue

Glycogen or animal starch is a complex carbohydrate that is the stored form of glucose (a source of energy) in animal cells. Glycogen is composed of branched chains of glucose units. Ultimately in metabolism, it is hydrolysed by enzymes to glucose. When glycogen is needed for energy, it is first converted to pyruvic acid according to the formula:

$$(C_6H_{11}O_5)n \longrightarrow CH_3-CO-COOH$$
$$\text{Pyruvic acid}$$

Excess glucose is stored as glycogen. Glycogen is found in the form of granules within specific cells. Hepatocytes have the highest concentration of glycogen. Muscle cells do not have a high concentration of glycogen but still have more than cells in the liver. Glycogen in the liver is used mostly as an energy reserve. Glycogen is found in small amounts in the kidneys and even smaller amounts in glial cells in the brain and in white blood cells. When glucose is abundant, glycogen is synthesized. When tissues need glucose, glycogen is broken down. Glycogen is stored in the liver tissue and can be measured by a characteristic reaction with iodine.

Hormones direct glycogen metabolism. Insulin directs the synthesis of glycogen. Glucagon directs the breakdown of glycogen primarily in the liver. Epinephrine directs the breakdown of glycogen mostly in muscle cells.

Experimental procedure

1. Remove the livers (or muscles) of 10-20 rats quickly and transfer as rapidly as possible to 300 ml. of 30% (w/v) NaOH at 100ºC.

2. Continue theheating for 2 hr. and then precipitate the crude glycogen by adding twice the volume of 96% (v/v) ethanol.

3. After separation, dissolve the precipitate in a small volume of water and adjust the pH to 3 with dilute HCI. Precipitate the glycogen by the addition of an equal volume of ethanol.

4. Repeat this process precipitation was repeated once more, and wash the resulting substance with ethanol and ether and finally dried in vacuo. Weigh the dry the powder.

Weigh of glycogen = ———— gm

Estimation of glycogen in the extract

It is estimated by using iodine reagent.

Iodine reagent

Prepare 16.5 ml. of Lugol's solution, by dissolving 1 gm of iodine and 2 gm of KI in 20 ml. of water. To this, add 990 ml. of an aqueous solution, containing 25% (w/v) of KCl.

Procedure

In a colorimeter tube (1.2 cm. diameter), mix 2 ml. of a liver extract and 3 ml of iodine reagent. After mixing, read the optical density in a photometer at 650 mmծ. against a blank, obtained by adding 2 ml. of 5% TCA to 3 ml. of reagent in the same way. Read the amount of glycogen from a calibration curve, which must be prepared using glycogen of the same origin as the sample to be estimated.

Note : Glycogen may also be estimated by using anthrone reagent.

Quantitative Determination of Glucose

Determination of glucose is based upon the presence of aldehydic group in glucose owing to which it reduces the Fehling solution (blue colour) into cuprous oxide (red colour). Fehling solution is obtained by mixing an aqueous copper sulphate solution (Fehling solution A) and alkaline solution of sodium potassium tartarate (Fehling solution B).

$$Cu(OH)_2 + C_6H_{12}O_6 \longrightarrow HOOC-(CHOH)_4-CH_2OH + Cu_2O$$

Glucose   Gluconic Acid   Cuprous Oxide

Experimental procedure

- Weigh accurately the sample (about 1.25 gm), dissolve in water and volume is make upto 250 ml in volumetric flask.
- Pipette out 25 ml of Fehling solution (Equal volume of Fehling A and B solution), dilute with water and boil gently over a gauze.
- Now titrate this solution with glucose solution untill blue color entirely dissappeared.
- Repeat the titrations untill consistent values are obtained.

According to theoretical concept, 1 ml of Fehling solution contain = 0.005 gm of pure glucose.

V (Titration reading) vol. of glucose solution contain = 25 × 0.005 gm of pure glucose.

$$\% \text{ of glucose} = \frac{25 \times 0.005 \times 250}{V \times Wt \text{ of sample}} \times 100$$

Fehling's solution A

Dissolve crystalline copper sulphate (17.32 gm) in water and make up the volume to 250 ml in volumetric flask

Fehling's solution B

Dissolve crystalline sodium potassium tartarate (86.5 gm) in warm water. Dissolve pure sodium hydroxide (30 gm) in water. Mix the tartarate and sodium hydroxide solution, cool and make up to 250 ml in volumetric flask.

When the Fehling's solution is required, transfer equal volumes of solution A and B to a dry flask and mix thoroughly by shaking.

11

Chemistry and Isolation of Starch from potato

Starch is a mixture of two complex carbohydrates: amylose and amylopectin, both of which are polymers of glucose. It is used by plants as a way to store excess glucose. The word is derived from Middle English *sterchen*, meaning to stiffen, which is appropriate since it can be used as a thickening agent when dissolved in water and heated.

The chemical formula for Starch is $(C_6H_{10}O_5)_n$, as it is a polymer of glucose. The chemical formula for glucose is $(C_6H_{12}O_6)$. In terms of human nutrition, starch is by far the most important of the polysaccharides. It constitutes more than half the carbohydrates even in many affluent diets, and much more in poorer diets. It is supplied by traditional staple foods such as cereals, roots and tubers.

Starch (in particular corn starch) is used in cooking for thickening foods such as sauce. In industry, it is used in the manufacturing of adhesives, paper, textiles and as a mold in the manufacture of sweets such as wine gums and jelly beans. It is a white powder, and depending on the source, may be tasteless and odourless.

Experimental procedure

(i) Wash potato(500gm) thoroughly with water to remove any oily particles.

(ii) Prepare a fine slurry with water in a blender.

(iii) Pass the slurry through a sieve with shaking to remove all debris and other impurities.

(iv) Allow the milky liquid to settle down.

(v) Decant the supernatant liquid. Wash starch 2-3 times with water.

(vi) Centrifuge in an oven at low temperature and grind.

(vii) Weigh the starch and report the yield.

Lipids

Contents

Experiment **12**

Introduction to Lipids

The lipids include not only true fats but substances chemically related to fats (like lecithin) or related to them because of common solubilities and possible biological relationship(like cholesterol). True fats and fixed oils are esters of glycerol and higher fatty acids. The classification of lipids includes:

1. Fats-esters of fatty acids and glycerol
2. Waxes- esters of fatty acids and certain alcohol

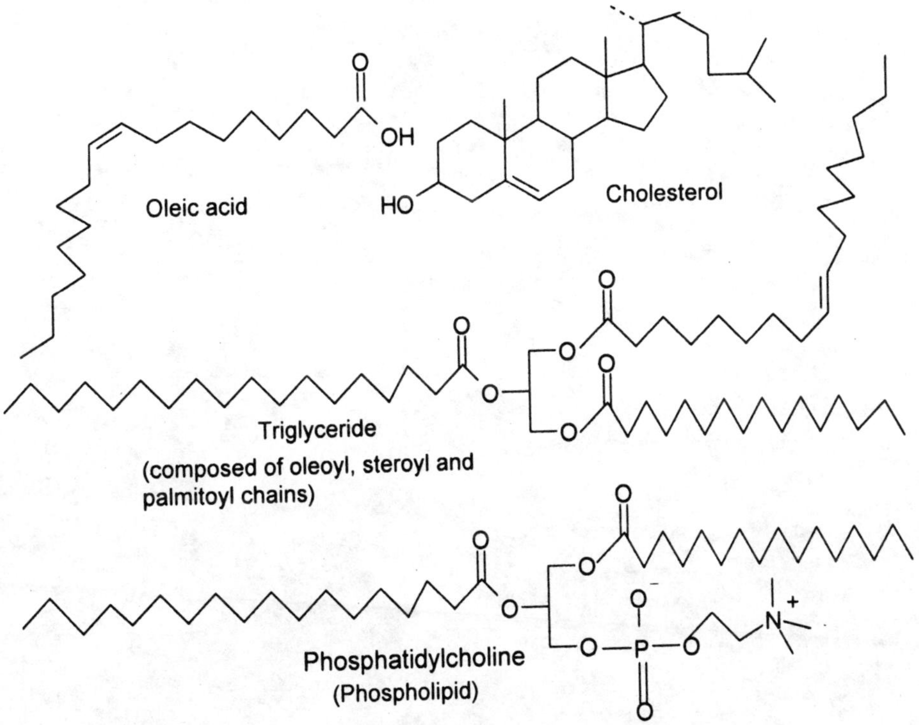
O
OH
Oleic acid
HO
Cholesterol
O
O
O
O
O
O
Triglyceride
(composed of oleoyl, steroyl and
palmitoyl chains)
O
O
O
O
O
O
P
O
O
N
+
Phosphatidylcholine
(Phospholipid)

3. Phospholipids- include phosphoric acid and nitrogen groups
4. Cerebrosides- fatty acids, sugars and nitrogenous groups
5. Sterols-hydrogenated phenanthrenes like ergosterol and cholesterol

The lipids are soluble generally in ether and other solvents whereas carbohydrates and proteins are practically insoluble in such solvents.

Lipid plays a diverse and important roles in nutrition and health. Many lipids are absolutely essential for life however, there is also considerable awareness that abnormal levels of certain lipids, particularly (in hypercholesteromia), and more recently, trans fatty acid, are risk factor for heart disease amongest other.

13

Tests for Lipids

Solubility in Polar and Nonpolar Solvents

Lipids are insoluble in polar solvents and soluble in non polar solvents. For this test, the polar solvent is water; the nonpolar solvent is corn oil:

1. Set up three tubes.
2. Add 1 ml (20 drops) each of the pair of liquids indicated below.
3. Mix the contents of each tube with mechanical shaking.
4. Wait for 2 minutes.
5. Lxamine each tube carefully. Has the sample dissolved in the solvent or do you see two separate layers in the tube?
6. Record your observations in Table I.
7. Save your tubes for the Sudan red test described below.

Table I. Results of Solubility Test and the Sudan Red Test for Lipids

Tube	Tubecontents	How many layers do you see? One or two?)	Is the second substancde soluble in water, a polar solvent	Is the second substance soluble in oil, a non-polar solvent?	Which layer does Sudan Red dissolve in and color red? (Water or oil?)
1	Water mixed with water				
2	Water mixed with corn oil				
3	Corn oil mixed with olive oil				

Sudan Red Test

Sudan red, dissolved in alcohol, is a lipid soluble dye. When Sudan red is added to a mixture of lipids and water, thc dye will move into the lipid layer coloring it red:

1. Add 5 drops of Sudan red dye to each tube from the solubility exercise described above, and

2. Mix the contents of each tube using the vortex genie.

3. Wait 2 minutes.

4. Examine each tube carefully. Where is the red color found?

"Grease Spot" Test

You perform this test every time you buy muffins or doughnuts in a paper bag. Lipids make unglazed paper (brown paper, writing paper) translucent:

1. Put a drop of each sample on a piece of unglazed paper.

2. Draw a circle around the spot with a soft pencil.

3. Write the name of the sample in pencil next to the spot.

4. Allow all spots to dry thoroughly.

5. Hold the paper in front of a light source and observe the spots.

6. Record your observations in Table II below.

Table II. Results of Grease Spot Test for Lipids in Foods

Spot number	Samples	Is the spot translucent? (Yes or no?)
	Standards:	
1	Water	
2	Corn Oil	
3	Olive oil	
	Do these foods contain lipids?	
4	Whole milk	
5	Skim milk	
6	Regular Soda	

Determination of acid value

Acid value is defined as the number of milligrams of potassium hydroxide required to neutralize the free fatty acids in one gram of an oil or fat. Acid value is a valuable test for freshness. Stale/rancid fats or oils have abnormally high acid value. Fats contain glycerides of fatty acid. Owing to liberation of free acid, a high acid value would be expected in a rancid fat.

Standard Values

Fat/oil	Acid Value	Fat/oil	Acid value
Lard oil	0.5 – 0.8	Cod liver oil	5.6
Seasame oil	9.8	Wool fat	59.8
Corn oil	1.37 – 2.02	Butter fat	0.4– 35.4
Castor oil	0.12 – 0.80	Olive oil	0.3 – 1.0
Cottonseed oil	0.6 – 0.9	Linseed oil	1 – 3.5
Palm oil	10		
Wax Acid Value			
Spermaceti	Below 1	Beeswax	18-24
Carnauba	4 – 7		

Determination of Acid Value (IP 1996 method)

Unless otherwise specified in the individual monograph, dissolve an accurately weighed quantity of the substance (10 gm) being examined in a mixture of equal volumes of 95% ethanol and ether (50 ml), previously neutralized with 0.1M potassium hydroxide solution to phenolphthalein solution. If the sample does not dissolve in the cold solvent, connect the flask with a reflux condenser and warm slowly, with frequent shaking, until the sample dissolved. Add phenolphthalein solution (1 ml) and titrate with 0.1M potassium hydroxide solution until the solution remains faintly pink after shaking for 30 seconds.

Note : If the oil has been saturated with carbon dioxide for the purpose of preservation gently reflux the solution of the oil in ethanol (95%) and ether for 10 minutes before titration. The oil may be freed from the carbon dioxide by exposing it in a shallow dish in a vacuum desicator for 24 hrs before weighing the sample.

Formula :

$$\text{Acid value} = \frac{5.61 \times n}{W}$$

where   n = Volume of Potassium hydroxide solution consumed.

   w = Weight (gm) of substance or the oil taken.

Determination of Saponification value

The saponification value of an oil or fat represents the number of mg of KOH needed to saponify 1gm of the substance. Roughly speaking, this varies with the molecular weight of the fat or oil. Some average accepted saponification values for common oils include:

Olive oil 185-196   Coconut oil 246-260

Linseed oil 192-195   Palm oil 242-250

Cottonseed oil 193-195   Peanut oil 188-195

Sesame oil 188-193   Corn oil 187-196

1. Saponification value is a measure of the size of the fat molecule or the size or molecular weight of fatty acids in the fat.

   (**Note:** Each molecule of fat regardless of its size requires three molecules of potassium hydroxide for saponification).

2. The saponification value indicates the quantity of alkali which must be used to convert a blend of fats to soap.

3. Saponification value is also useful for detecting adulteration of a given fat by one of the higher or lower saponification value.

Experimental procedure

Place 2 gm of one of the oils above in a 250 ml flask and add 25ml of a 0.5N alcoholic KOH solution. Heat the flask under refluxing condition for 45 minutes. Then add 1ml of phenolphthalein and titrate the excess of KOH with 0.5N HCl. Now run a blank test, using exactly the same amount of 0.5N alcoholic KOH. The difference between the number of ml of 0.5N HCl consumed in the actual test and in the blank test multiplied by 28.05 is the saponification value of the oil being tested. Run two more oil samples through this procedure and record result.

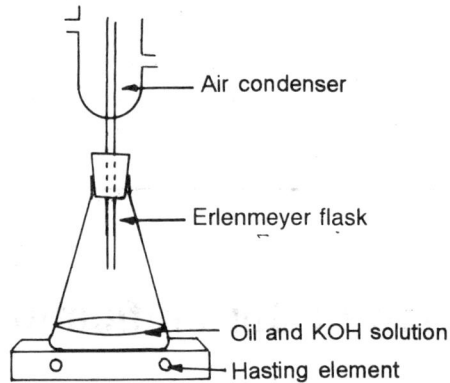

Air condenser

Erlenmeyer flask

Oil and KOH solution

Hasting element

Fig. 15.1. Detm of Saponification value

1. ml HCl used in first oil test – ml HCl in blank × 28.05 saponification number of first oil
2. ml HCl used in second oil test – ml HCl in blank × 28.05 saponification number of second oil
3. ml HCl used in third oil test – ml HCl in blank × 28.05 saponification number of third oil

Similarly, the ester value of these sample can be determined.

Ester value : Saponification value – Acid value

Iodine value

The iodine value of a fat or oil represents the number of grams of iodine absorbed under the prescribed conditions by 100 gm of the oil or fat. Iodine value is regarded as a measure of its degree of unsaturation and gives an idea of its drying characters. A high IV oil contains a greater number of double bonds than a low IV oil. Edible oils with high iodine value are usually less stable. Iodine value is also helpful in finding adulteration in fats and oils and judging its suitability in paint industry. The iodine numbers of some common oils are as follows:

Olive oil	79-88	Seasame oil	103-122
Linseed oil	173-201	Corn oil	109-133
Cottonseed oil	108-110	Peanut oil	84-104
Coconut oil	8-10	Soybean oil	127-138
Palm oil	13-17	Safflower oil	140-150

Determination of Iodine Value of oil/fat

Iodine value is determined by the following methods:

1. Iodine Monochloride Method or Wij's Method:

This method was devised by Wij. It uses the solution of iodine monochloride in a mixture of carbon tetrachloride and glacial acetic acid. Fats or oils due to presence of double bonds combines with iodine and the result is calculated as equivalent to iodine.

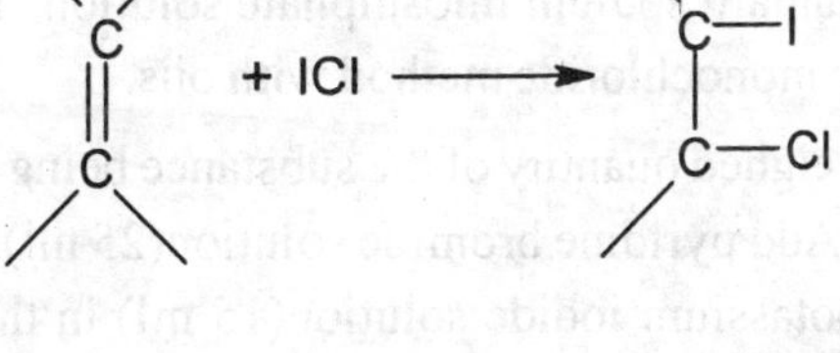

41

Dissolve an accurately weighed quantity of the substance being examined in a dry 500 ml iodine flask in carbon tetrachloride (10 ml). Add of iodine monochloride solution(20 ml), and allow to stand in the dark at a temperature between 15° and 25°C for 30 minutes. Introduce potassium iodide solution(15 ml) in the cuptop. Carefully remove the stopper, rinse the stopper and the sides of the flask with water(100 ml). Shake and titrate with 0.1M sodium thiosulphate solution using starch solution as indicator.Similarly carry out the blank titration.

Formula :

$$\text{Iodine value} = \frac{(b - a) \times 1.269}{\text{Weight of sample}}$$

where   b = Volume of Sod. thiosulphate solution consumed in blank titration

a = Volume of Sod. thiosulphate solution consumed in sample titration

Note: The approximate weight in 'gm' of a substance to be taken may be calculated by dividing 20 by the highest expected iodine value. If more than half the available halogen is absorbed, the test must be repeated with smaller amount of the substance(oil/fat).

There are two ways for preparing Wij's solution:

(a) Chlorine is passed through a solution of iodine in a mixture of carbon tetrachloride and glacial acetic acid. The completion of reaction is completed as shown by the titre value of solution with sodium thiosulphate, after the addition of potassium iodide.

$$Cl_2 + I_2 \longrightarrow 2ICl$$
$$ICl + KI \rightleftharpoons KCl + I_2$$

(b) Interaction of iodine trichloride in glacial acetic acid with iodine in carbon tetrachloride yield iodine monochloride.The mixture is then diluted with glacial acetic acid.

$$I_2 + ICl_3 \rightleftharpoons ICl$$

2. Pyridne Bromide Method

This method makes use of additive compound of pyridine bromide and sulphuric acid. This reagent forms additive compound with unsaturated glyceride without any substitution or oxidation and the excess of pyridine bromide can subsequently be determined by the addition of potassium iodide followed by titration with standard sodium thiosulphate solution. This method is said to give more consistent results then iodine monochloride method with oils.

Dissolve an accurately weighed quantity of the substance being examined in a dry iodine flask in carbon tetrachloride(10 ml). Add pyridine bromide solution(25 ml), allow to stand for 10 minutes in the dark and transfer 10% potassium iodide solution(15 ml) in the cuptop. Carefully remove the stopper, rinse the stopper and sides of the flask with water (100 ml), shake and titrate with 0.1M sodium thiosulphate solution using starch solution as indicator, towards the end of the titration. Similarly carry out the blank titration.

Formula :

$$\text{Iodine value} = \frac{(b-a) \times 1.269}{\text{Weight of sample}}$$

where   b = Volume of Sod. thiosulphate solution consumed in blank titration

a = Volume of Sod. thiosulphate solution consumed in sample titration

Note: The approximate weight in gm, of the substance to be taken may be calculated by dividing 12.5 by the highest expected value. If more than half the available halogen is absorbed, the test must be repeated with smaller quantity of substance.

Pyridine bromide Solution

Dissolve pyridine (8 gm) and sulphuric acid (5.4 ml) in glacial acetic Keeping the mixture cool, add bromine solution (2.6 ml dissolved in glacial acetic acid (20 ml) and then dilute the solution to 1000 ml with acetic acid.

Note: The above two methods are official in I P1996.

Determination of R M and Polenske values

The soluble volatile fatty acid value (Reichert or Reichert-Meissl-Wollny-value, R.M. value) is the number of millilitres of aqueous 0.1 N alkali solution required to neutralize the water soluble volatile fatty acids obtained from 5 grammes of fat under the specific conditions of the method.

The insoluble volatile fatty acid value (Polenske value) is the number of millilitres of acqueous 0.1 N alkali solution required to neutralize the water insoluble volatile fatty acids obtained from 5 gm of fat under the specific conditions of the method.

Principle

After saponification of the fat with sodium hydroxide solution in glycerol, the soap solution is diluted with water and acidified with sulphuric acid. The volatile fatty acids are distilled and the insoluble fatty acids are separated from the soluble acids by filtration. The aqueous solution of the soluble acids and the ethanolic solution of the insoluble acids are then titrated separately with a standardized alkali solution.

The method is empirical for it determines only a part of these acids. Consequently, the specifications for procedure and apparatus must be followed rigorously in order to obtain accurate and reproducible results.

Reagents

Glycerol (d = 1.26; 98 % w/w)

Aqueous sodium hydroxide solution (44 % w/w), stored in a bottle protected from carbon dioxide. Use the clear portion free from carbonate deposit.

Distilled water freed from carbon dioxide by boiling for 15 minutes.

Sulphuric acid solution (1 N).

Aqueous sodium or potassium hydroxide solution (0.1 N) accurately standardized.

Phenolphthalein indicator solution (1 % in 95–96 % ethanol).

Ethanol (95–96 % v/v). neutral to phenolphthalein.

All reagents shall be of analytical grade. Water used should be distilled water or water of at least equal purity.

Procedure

Determination of soluble volatile fatty acid value

Weigh 5.00 ± 0.01 gm of the fat into the flask. Add 20 gm (16 ml) of glycerol and 2 ml of the sodium hydroxide solution (44 %).

Note : For supplying the sodium hydroxide solution, use a burette protected from the entry of carbon dioxide and clean the burette jet by rejecting the first few drops from the tap.

Heat the flask over a naked flame, avoiding overheating and shaking continuously until the liquid no longer foams and becomes clear.

Allow the flask to cool to about 90°C, add 90 ml of recently boiled distilled water of about the same temperature and mix. The liquid should remain clear. Add 0.6 to 0.7 gm of the pumice and then 50 ml sulphuric acid solution (1 N).

Connect the flask immediately to the distillation apparatus and warm it gently until the free fatty acids form a clear surface layer.

Start heating and regulate the flame so as to collect in the measuring flask 110 ml of distillate in 19–21 min., taking the moment when the first drop forms in the condenser as the beginning of the distillation period. Regulate the water flowing in the condenser so as to maintain the temperature of the water leaving the condenser at 20 ± 1°C.

When exactly 110 ml of distillate have been collected, remove the burner immediately and substitute a small beaker for the measuring flask.

Mix the contents of the measuring flask by gentle shaking and immerse the flask in a waterbath at 20 ± 1°C for 10 to 15 minutes, the 110 ml mark on the flask being 1 cm below the level of the water in the waterbath and the flask being turned from time to time.

Stopper the flask and mix by inverting it 4 to 5 times without shaking.

Filter the 110 ml of distillate through a dry medium speed filter paper (diameter 80–90 mm) which fits snugly into the funnel. The filtrate should be clear.

Pipette 100 ml of the filtrate into a conical flask of 300 ml, add 0.5 ml of phenolphthalein indicator solution and titrate with the standardized aqueous alkali solution (0.1 N) to a pink colour persistent for 1/2 to 1 minute.

Blank test

Conduct a blank test without fat and instead of saponifying over a naked flame, heat over a boiling water bath for 15 minutes.

Note : Not more than 0.5 ml of the standardized alkali solution should be required for the titration. Otherwise, new reagent solutions should be prepared.

Determination of insoluble volatile fatty acid value

Rinse the filter with three successive 15 ml portions of distilled water at a temperature of $20 \pm 1°C$, each having previously passed through the condenser, the small beaker and the measuring flask.

Place the funnel and filter in the neck of a dry clean conical flask of 200 ml capacity.

Dissolve the insoluble fatty acids by repeating the washing procedure using now 15 ml of ethanol (95–96 %).

Titrate the combined ethanolic washings with the standardized aqueous alkali solution (0.1 N), using 0.5 ml of phenolphthalein indicator solution, to a pink colour persistent for 1/2 to 1 min.

Calculation

Soluble volatile fatty acid value (R.M. value)

Reichert value = 11.t. $(v_1 - b)$

where

v_1 = number of millilitres standardized alkali solution (0.1 N) required for the sample

b = number of millilitres standardized alkali solution (0.1 N) required for the blank test

t = exact normality of the standardized alkali solution (0.1 N).

Report the result rounded to the first decimal place.

Insoluble volatile fatty acid value (Polenske value)

Polenske value = 10.t.v_2

where v_2 = number of ml standardized alkali solution (0.1 N) required for the sample

t = exact normality of the standardized alkali solution (0.1 N).

Report the result rounded to the first decimal place.

Repeatability of results

The difference between results of duplicate determinations (results obtained simultaneously or in rapid succession by the same analyst) should not exeed 0.5 for the Reichert value and 0.3 for the Polenske value

Isolation of Cholesterol from Gallstones

Cholesterol is an example of the steroid class of lipids that are characterized by a cyclopentano-perhydrophenanthrene ring system. It occurs in brain tissue, gallstones and blood. Its structure is:

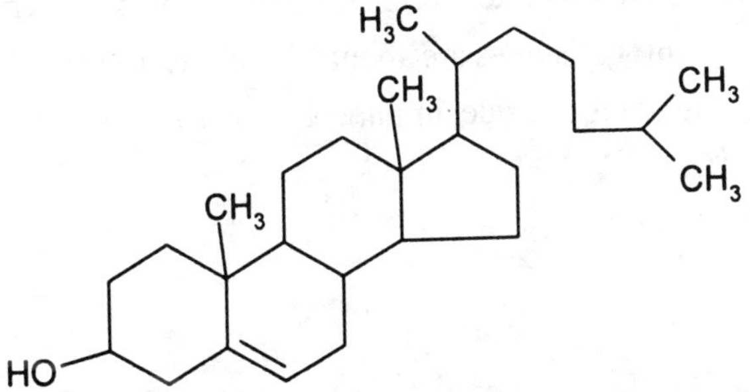

For isolation, weigh 8 gm of pulverized gallstones and place them in 125 ml flask. Add 40ml of diethyl ether and heat the mixture on a steam bath until the cholesterol is dissolved. Filter the brownish yellow solution through a funnel while it is still hot and add a little ether to replace that lost through evaporation. The brown residue that collects on the filter paper is bilirubin, a bile pigment derived from hemoglobin with the structure:

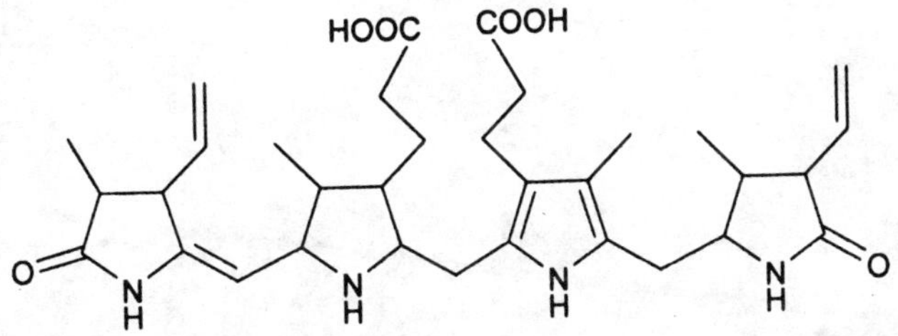

Dilute this filtrate with 40 ml methanol, add a little decolorizing agent and heat the mixture on a steam bath. Preheat a funnel, then filter the hot solution through this funnel. Reheat the greenish yellow filtrate and add just enough water, dropwise to make the solution cloudy. The solution is now saturated at the boiling and cholesterol will crystallize upon cooling. Collect the crystals by vacuum filtration using a small Buchner funnel as shown in the diagram.

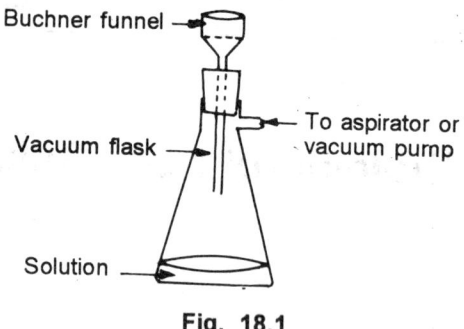

Buchner funnel

To aspirator or vacuum pump

Vacuum flask

Solution

Fig. 18.1

Wash the crystals with cold methanol and allow them to stand for a time in the open Buchner funnel to allow the solvent to evaporate. Weigh the dried cholesterol crystals

Result: ——— gm(Hint: gallstones are about 60% cholesterol).

Determine the melting point of crude, impure cholesterol

Result: ——— °C.

Some Color Reactions of Cholesterol

A number of time-honored tests can be run with cholesterol sample isolated from the previous experiment which include the iodine-sulphuric test, the Salkowski reaction, the Libermann-Burchard reaction, and the Rosenheim trichloroacetic test. These are also reffered as general test for steroid nucleus containing substance.

Iodine-sulphuric Acid test

Prepare a mixture of 10ml concentrated H_2SO_4, and 2 ml H_2O. Mix well and allow to cool. Evaporate to dryness in test tube 1ml of 0.1% cholesterol in chloroform. After the chloroform is removed completely and the tubes have cooled, add 5ml of the above prepared H_2SO_4 solution. Record result for color change. Now add 1drop of 0.1N I_2 in KI and record result.

Add 2 drops more of the Iodine/KI reagent and record result.

Salkowski reaction

Place 1ml of 1% Cholesterol solution in test tube and add 1ml of concentrated sulphuric acid to it. *Cholesterol will shows the yellow ring at the junction which turns red after one minute.*

Liebermann-Burchard Reaction

This teaction is used for the quantitative estimation of cholesterol. Place 1ml of a 0.1% solution of cholesterol in chloroform. Add 5drops of acetic anhydride to this. Mix well and add 1 drop of concentrated H_2SO_4 to it. Note the color changes and intensities for the first 5 minutes. *Blue or red color is produced.*

Rosenheim trichloroacetic acid

To 1ml of the 0.1% cholesterol in chloroform, add 1 ml of trichloroacetic acid solution(9:1 mix of $TCA:H_2O$) and record result.

Estimation of Cholesterol content by Liebermann-Burchard method

Cholesterol is the most abundant sterol in animal tissues. It is a derivative of saturated tetracyclic hydrocarbon-perhydro cyclopentenophenanthre ring.

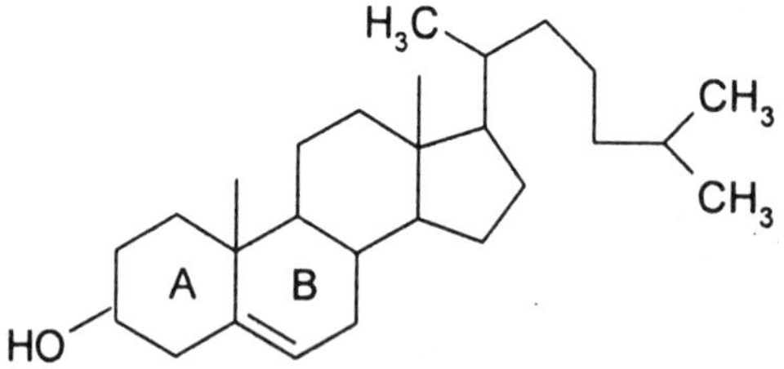

Cholesterol

Blood cholesterol value is an important diagnostic parameter from clinical point of view. The libermann-Burchard test is based on the fact that the sterols with unsaturation in the ring B react with sulphuric acid in the presence of acetic anhydride to give blue color which immediately changes to green. During the reaction, dehydration, condensationand isomerisation take place with the formation of chromophoric salt which is green in color. The exact nature of the chromophore is not known but reaction includes esterification of the hydroxyl group at position 3 and sterols become activated and green color is produced due to shift in double bond.

Method

For preparation of standard color, pipette out solution containing 10-100 mg cholesterol in different test tubes and make the volume to 1ml with chloroform. Take a suitable volume of the extract in which cholesterol has to be estimated and make its volume up to 1 ml. *[Blood or serum is extracted with an alcohol-acetone(1:1) mixture which removes cholesterol and other lipids and precipitates protein. The organic solvent is removed by evaporation on a boiling water bath*

50

and dry residue dissolved in chloroform]. Add 5 ml of acetic anhydride-sulphuric acid mixture (30:1, v/v) carefully to each test tube. Mix well and not the change in color of the solution. Cover the test tubes and leave them in dark for 15 minutes.

Measure the absorbance of the solution at 640nm and draw the standard curve for cholesterol. From the standard curve, calculate the amount of cholesterol present in 1ml of the sample preparation.

Precautions

1. All the apparatus used for this experiment should be absolutely dry.
2. Acetic anhydride and sulphuric acid reagent should be colorless.

vial is full. If the yellow band is not finished when the vial is full, continue to collect the yellow band in vial #2, 3, etc. When the yellow band is out of the column, collect any clear solvent in your

Proteins

Contents

Introduction to proteins

Proteins belong to a group of one of the most complex of chemical substances. They are essential constituents of all protoplasm as well as being an essential food constituent. These are classified as:-

1. Simple proteins

Albumins are soluble in water and in dilute salt solution and include egg white and serum albumin.

Globulins are insoluble in all neutral solvents but soluble in dilute solutions of acids and bases and include egg yolk, fibrinogens of blood, and myosin of muscle.

Prolamins are insoluble in water but soluble in 70% alcohol and include gliadin of

Albuminoids are insoluble in all neutral solvents and include keratin of horns and hair and elastin of ligaments.

Histones are soluble in water and dilute acids but insoluble in dilute NH_3 and include globin from blood hemoglobin.

Protamines are soluble in NH_3 and water and uncoagulable by heat and are present in salmon and sturgeon sperm.

2. Conjugated proteins

Nucleoproteins, on hydrolysis yield protein and nucleic acid and are present in glandular tissue and yeast.

Glycoproteins are proteins combined with a carbohydrate group and include mucin of saliva.

Phosphoproteins contain phosphoric acid combined with amino groups and include casein of milk and vitellin of egg yolk.

Lecithoproteins are proteins combined with lecithin and are found in tissue fibrinogens.

3. Derived proteins

Proteans are products of enzymatic digestion of globulins, soluble in weak acids and bases, including edestan and myosin

Metaproteins are soluble in weak acids and base but insoluble in neutral water and include acid albuminate and alkali albuminate.

Coagulated proteins are water insoluble resulting from action of heat, alcohol, heavy metal salts and X-rays on proteins

Proteoses are soluble in water and not coaguable by heat and are precipitated by solutions of ammonium sulphate.

Peptones are soluble in water and are not precipitated by ammonium sulphate and are not coaguable by heat.

Peptides are combinations of two or more amino acids joined by the peptide linkage.

Proteins are complex substances of high molecular weight that, on hydrolysis yield amino acids in addition to other products of decomposition, the character and quality of which vary with different kinds of proteins. The hydrolytic changes are produced by acids, bases, water and specific enzymes. Proteins are polymers of amino acid just as polysaccharides are polymers of monosaccharides. The linking unit between terminals of amino acids is called a peptide bond.

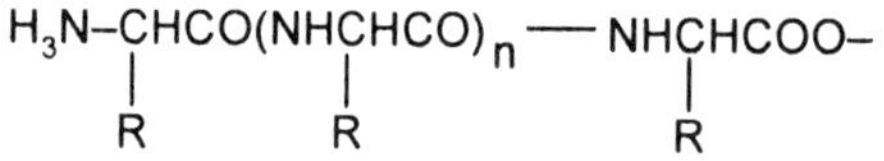

$$H_3N-\underset{\underset{R}{|}}{C}HCO(NH\underset{\underset{R}{|}}{C}HCO)_n \longrightarrow NH\underset{\underset{R}{|}}{C}HCOO-$$

Some Color Reactions of Proteins

Biuret reaction

To 2 ml of a protein, add 2ml of a 10% NaOH solution and 1drop of 1% $CuSO_4$ solution Mix well. Pink to Violet color is produced. Be careful not to put in excess copper, since an excess combined with protein substances, obscures the true color.

Biuret is obtained by heating urea. Biuret contains amide bonds similar to those in proteins. Biuret reacts with copper (II) ions (blue) in basic solution to form a purple complex ion. This test is given by all proteins that contain two or more peptide linkages.

$$2H_2N-CO-NH_2 \longrightarrow H_2N-CONH-CO-NH_2 + NH_3$$

Urea   Biuret

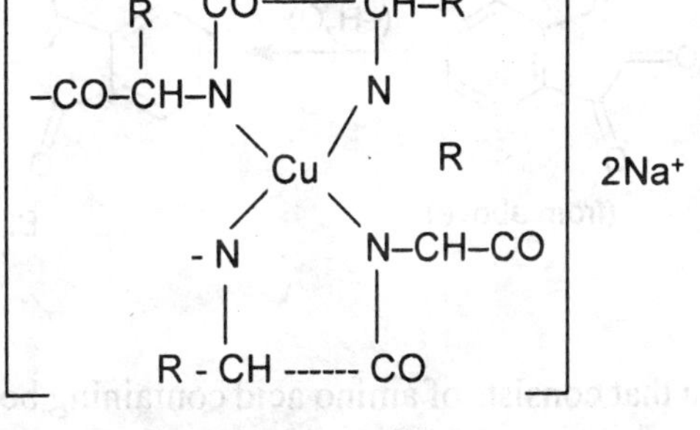

Colored Complex

A deep violet or blue color indicates the presence of proteins and a light pink color indicates the presence of peptides.

Biuret Reagent : Add, with stirring, 300 mL of 10% (w/v) NaOH to 500 ml of a solution containing 0.3% copper sulphate pentahydrate and 1.2% sodium potassium tartrate, then dilute to one liter. The reagent is stable for a few months but not a year. Adding one gram of potassium iodide per liter and storing in the dark makes it stable indefinitely.

Ninhydrin reaction

Ninhydrin, which is chemically is triketohydrindene hydrate, reacts very delicately in detecting not only proteins and amino acids but very sensitive to pH.

To a 2 ml protein solution, add 1ml of 0.1% ninhydrin solution and boil for one minute. A violet color is produced.

The ninhydrin reaction is used to detect the presence of α-amino acids and proteins containing free amino groups. When heated with ninhydrin, these molecules give characteristic deep blue colours (or occasionally pale yellow). The reactions involved in this test are shown below.

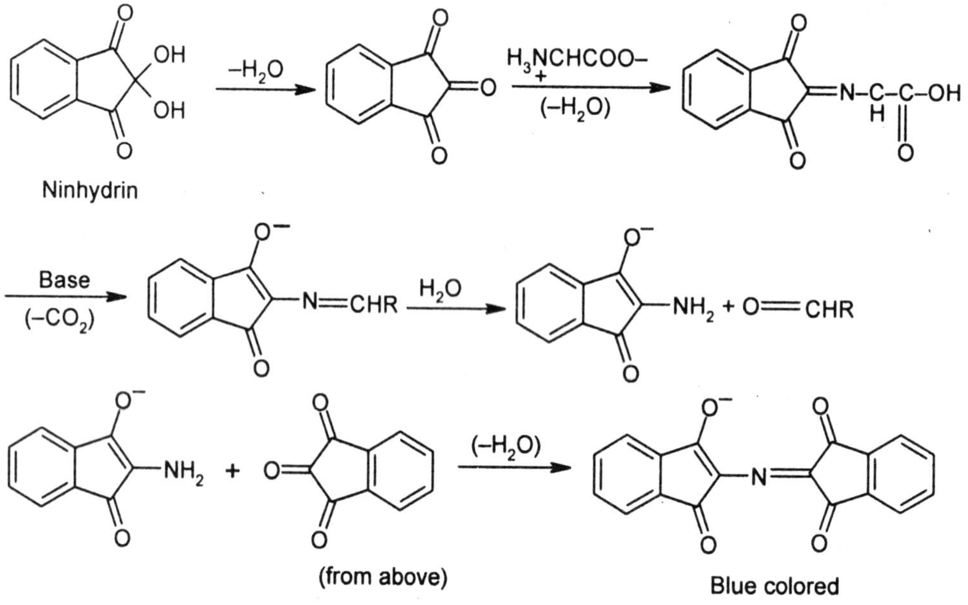

Ninhydrin

(from above)   Blue colored

Xanthoproteic reaction

This test is given by a protein that consists of amino acid containing benzene nucleus. This reaction involves the nitration of the benzene nucleus and resulting color when the solution is rendered alkaline.

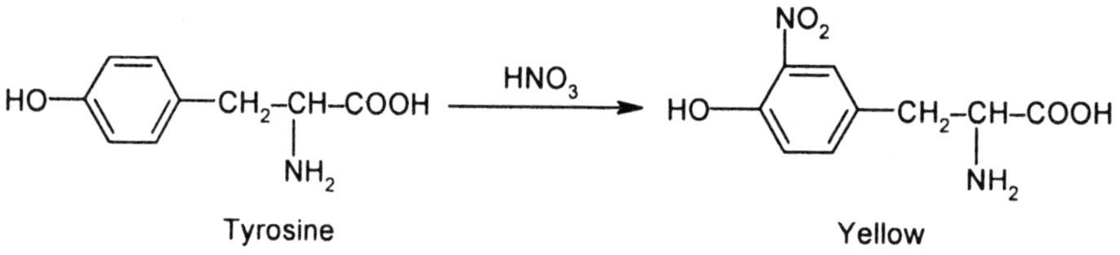

Tyrosine   Yellow

To a few mg of tyrosine, tryptophan and phenylalanine in four small test tubes, add 1 ml of conc. HNO_3 to each tube and boil until the amino acids are dissolved. Now cool and add a few drops of 40% NaOH solution until the solution is slightly alkaline as determined by litmus paper. Observe the change in coloration. *A yellow color is produced.*

Millon's reaction

The Millon's reagent consists of mercury dissolved in nitric acid (forming a mixture of mercuric and mercurous nitrates and nitrites).

To 3ml of a solution of tyrosine, add several drops of Millon's reagent, yellow color is produced.

*Millon's test is given by any compound containing a phenolic hydroxy group. Consequently, any protein containing tyrosine will give a positive test of a pink to dark-red color. (**Caution: Million's reagent is highly toxic and highly corrosive**). The red colour is probably due to a mercury salt of nitrated tyrosine. The presence of Cl^- or NH_4^+ ions interfere with this reaction. You should rinse the test tube with deionized water before performing this test.*

Hopkins-Cole reaction

Add concentrated H_2SO_4 down the side of a test tube containing a solution of protein and glyoxalic acid to form a layer. A violet ring appears at the junction. *This reaction is given by protein which have the amino acid, tryptophan in its structure.*

Sulphur Test

Cysteine and methionine are the sulphur containing amino acids, but differ in that cysteine can be oxidized in alkaline solution to form a disulphide bond linking two molecules to form cystine, which reacts with lead, while methionine has a methyl group on the sulphur making it less reactive toward lead.

The presence of sulphur-containing amino acids such as cysteine can be determined by converting the sulphur to an inorganic sulphide through cleavage by base. When the resulting solution is combined with lead acetate, a black precipitate of lead sulphide results.

$$\text{Sulfur-containing protein} \xrightarrow{\text{NaOH}} S^{2-} - Pb^{2+} \longrightarrow PbS\downarrow$$
$$\text{black precipitate}$$

Place 1 mL of casein, 2% egg albumin, and 0.1 M cysteine into separate, test tubes. Add 2 mL of 10% aqueous Sodium hydroxide followed by lead acetate solution and observe the color of precipitates.

Preparation of Casein from skimmed Milk

The proteins of milk include casein, lactaalbumin, and lactoglobulin, with casein comprising about 80% of the total protein. Casein is a phosphoprotein which yield phosphoric acid and amino acids on hydrolysis. The isoelectric point of casein is a pH of about 4.6 but the pH of milk is about 7.0, thus indicating that the casein in milk is in alkaline combination, probably in the form of calcium casein.

Casein is insoluble in water. The addition of acids to milk serves to precipitate it. The casein precipitated can be redissolved in an alkaline solution and then reprecipitated by acids, thus serving as a method of purifying the protein.

$$\text{Na caseinate} + \text{HCl} \longrightarrow \text{NaCl} + \text{H caseinate (or casein)}$$

$$\text{Casein hydrate} + \text{HCl} \longrightarrow \text{Casein} + \text{H}_2\text{O}$$

The preparation process

To 100 ml of skimmed milk in a 1000 ml beaker, add 300 ml of H_2O. Mix well and remove 40 ml of the mixture to a small beaker and add, carefully, drop a 10% H_2SO_4 solution, to get a coarsely flocculent precipitate of casein. Now return the 40ml to the larger sample of diluted milk and, in the same way, drop by drop add 10% H_2SO_4 in the same ratio while constantly stirring.

Be very careful not to add the acid too fast, as you miss the critical point and casein will redissolve to form casein sulphate. If this happen, you may add some 10% NaOH solution until the casein reprecipitates. To the crude casein, add 30 ml of water and stir until the precipitate is finely divided. To this suspension now add gradually a 10% solution of NaOH and stir until all the precipitate has now dissolved.

The next step is to reprecipitate the casein by slowly adding 10% acetic acid solution. After achieving a good coarse flocculent precipitate, decant the supernatant and wash the precipitate with 300ml of distilled water several times.

Finally, transfer the precipitate to a Buchner funnel, filter, and suction dry by vacuum. Remove the casein from the funnel, place in a mortar, and gradually add 50ml of ethanol while kneading the powder. Again filter by suction. Repeat this process two more times and finally dry.

After the casein is thouroghly dry, enter your result below:

Weight of 1000 ml beaker and 100 ml milk —————

Weight of 1000 ml beaker (minus) —————

Weight of 100 ml milk —————

Weight of casein precipitate —————

$$\% \text{ composition of casein} = \frac{\text{Weight of casein}}{\text{Weight of milk}} \times 100 = \text{.......}\%$$

Preparation of Edestin from Hemp Seed

Edestin is a protein present in hemp, commonly called marijuana, or botanically known as *Cannabis sativa*. The seeds contain some fats that must be extracted by the use of a suitable fat solvent.

To do this, begin by thoroughly grinding the seed in a mortar then transfer to a small flask and cover with a layer of benzene. Stopper the flask and place on a magnetic stirrer to agitate overnight. Filter this by gravity, dispose of the filtrate, and repeat the procedure with the seeds. Then expose the seeds and solvent on a watch glass and allow all solvents to evaporate. Caution: donot use any flames

To 10 gm of the finally ground fat-free hemp, add 100 ml of a 1%NaCl solution in a 250 ml flask. Place in a water bath maintained at 60°C for 1 hour. Do not allow the temperature to go above this number as it will cause the edestin to coagulate. Now filter the warm solution until you have collected about 75 ml of filtrate. This should be slightly turbid due to the separation of the edestin. Warm this filtrate in a warm bath again at 60°C until clear.

Once the solution is clear, discontinue heating and allow the flask to remain in the water overnight. This effects a slow cooling process, which results in the formation of larger crystals of edestin being formed than if the cooling were done more rapidly.

Filter the edestin crystal and perform % calculation as follows:

$$\frac{\text{Weight of edestin obtained}}{\text{Weight of hemp speed}} \times 100 = \ldots\ldots\%$$

Isolation of Cystine from Human Hair

Cystine may be obtained by the hydrolysis of a large number of proteins. However, the keratins are only common protein rich enough in cystine to serve as a source of this amine acid.

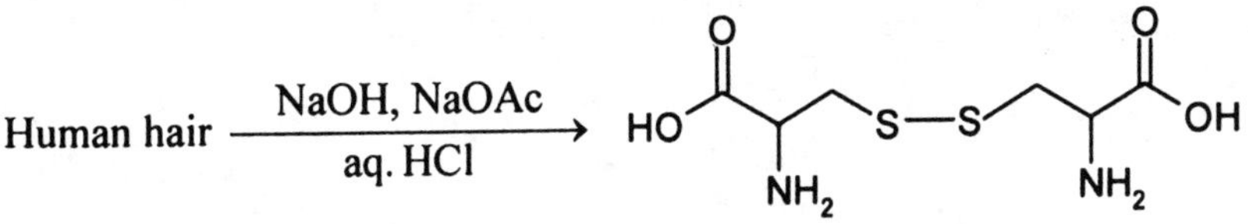

$$\text{Human hair} \xrightarrow[\text{aq. HCl}]{\text{NaOH, NaOAc}} $$

Cystine

Requirements

Human hair	= 250 gm
Sodium hydroxide solution	= sufficient quantity
Conc. HCl	= sufficient quantity

Procedure

Add thoroughly clean and dry hair in portion of 50 gm to concentrated hydrochloric acid (500 ml) in a round bottom flask. Heat under refluxing condition for 5–6 hrs until a drop of it no longer gives violet color with alkaline copper sulphate solution (Biuret reaction). Partially neutralize the solution in hot condition with a sodium hydroxide solution and then add sufficient sodium acetate solution. The Congo red litmus paper test for mineral acid should then be entirely negative at this stage. Care must be taken not to make the solution alkaline with NaOH*. Allow the contents to rest overnight and filter

---

* An alkaline reaction must always be avoided, as even dilute sodium carbonate decomposes cystine. For this reason, some have even preferred to omit the partial neutralization with NaOH and to employ sodium acetate only.

it to get brown colored precipitate which in addition to cystine also contain some "human" pigments and tyrosine. Transfer the precipitate to beaker and add hydrochloric acid (about 150 ml).boil and filter. Add a further hydrochloric acid (150 ml), boil and filter. To the hot clear filtrate, add concentrated solution of sodium acetate until Congo red paper reaction is negative and then cool in ice bath when Cystine separates as colorless crystalline powder. Filter the cystine and wash with hot distilled (in portion) and dry. Do not allow the filtrate to stand for a longer time, otherwise tyrosine may also crystallize out.

Calculate the % yield.

Paper Chromatography of Amino Acids

Proteins can be hydrolysed in acidic or basic solution or with enzymes causing the peptide bonds to give shorter polypeptides, which in turn are further degrade to amino acids. Total hydrolysis of proteins can be achieved in 20% HCl at 100°C for 12 to 48 hours. However, adequate hydrolysis for purposes of this experiment can be achieved in less than 1 hr.

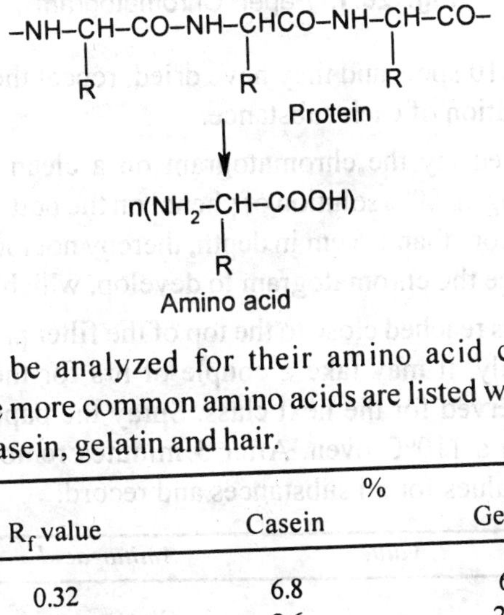

$$-NH-CH-CO-NH-CHCO-NH-CH-CO-$$

$$\underset{R}{|} \qquad \underset{R}{|} \qquad \underset{R}{|}$$

Protein

$$\downarrow$$

$$n(NH_2-CH-COOH)$$

$$\underset{R}{|}$$

Amino acid

These hydrolsates can be analyzed for their amino acid content by methods such as chromatography. Some of the more common amino acids are listed with their approximate R_f values and their % composition in casein, gelatin and hair.

| Amino acid | R_f value | % | | |
		Casein	Gelatin	Hair
Aspartic acid	0.32	6.8	6.7	3.9
Glutamic acid	0.40	2.6	25.5	4.1
Threonine	0.51	4.7	1.9	8.5
Alanine	0.59	2.9	8.7	2.8
Tyrosine	0.62	6.1	0.4	2.2
Valine	0.75	6.9	2.5	5.5
Leucine	0.79	8.8	4.6	11.2
Phenylalanine	0.82	4.8	2.2	2.4
Proline	0.85	10.9	18.0	4.3

Paper Chromatography Procedure

Using a 24 × 15.5 cm rectangle of filter paper (be careful not to touch anything but the edges of the paper or a false chromatogram may be given), pencil a line across the bottom about 2 cm from the edge. Then about 2 cm apart, make pencil dots for 10 equally spaced where you will apply the various solutions. In the first seven spots, You will pipet a dot 1-2 mm in diameter of 0.1M solution of aspartic acid, glutamic acid, threonine, alanine, valine, leucine, and praline, and in the last three spots you will pipet 1-2 mm diameter dots of the hydrolysates of casein, gelatin, and hair. Each of these solutions should have been acidified with 10 drops of 19% HCl for each 10 ml of solution.

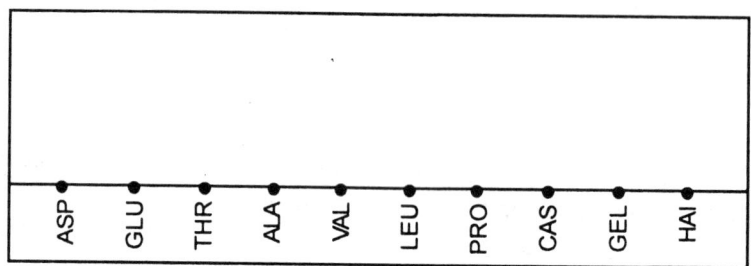

Fig. 26.1. Paper Chromatogram.

Once you have made the 10 spots and they have dried, repeat the pipet procedure to make sure you have sufficient concentration of each substance.

Once the spots have dried lay the chromatogram on a clean sheet of paper and prepare a developing chamber by placing an 80% solution of phenol on the bottom of a 2000 ml beaker, making sure that it does not become more than 1.5 cm in depth, thereby not touching your amino acid spot on the chromatogram. Now, place the chromatogram to develop, which should take a couple of hours.

When the phenol front has reached close to the top of the filter paper, you should remove it with a tweezers and dry thoroughly. It may take a couple of hrs for the solvent to evaporate, so the spraying session may be reserved for the next class. Spray the paper uniformly with a ninhydrin spray and place the paper in a 110°C oven. After 5 minutes remove the paper and observe the colored spots. Calculate R_f values for all substances and record:

Amino acid	R_f value	Amino acid	R_f value
Aspartic acid	–	Glutamic acid	–
Threonine	–	Alanine	–
Valine	–	Leucine	–
Proline	–	Casein	–
Gelatin	–	Hair	–

27

Total Protein Estimation by Lowry's Method

This was the chemical method most extensively used by biochemists over the past 50 years for estimation of the concentration of a protein in solution. A blue color is produced in a biuret reaction when the protein reacts with Cu^{2+} ions in a basic solution. The intensity of the color is enhanced by the reduction of a phosphomolybdic-phosphotungstic reagent by tyrosine and tryptophan amino acid side chains of the protein and its absorbance is measured at 500 nm. Several reagents interfere with the Lowry procedure, it requires several reagents added sequentially and it takes longer for the color to develop then the Bradford method. Many labs have switched from the Lowry method but the Lowry is still a very common protein assay technique. Like the Bradford procedure a standard curve must be prepared when the Lowry method is used.

Principle

The phenolic group of tyrosine and trytophan residues (amino acid) in a protein will produce a blue purple color complex , with maximum absorption in the region of 660 nm wavelength, with Folin-Ciocalteau reagent which consists of sodium tungstate, molybdate and phosphate. Thus the intensity of color depends on the amount of these aromatic amino acids present and will thus vary for different proteins. Most proteins estimation techniques use **Bovin Serum Albumin** (BSA) universally as a standard protein, because of its low cost, high purity and ready availability. The method is sensitive down to about 10 µg/ml and is probably the most widely used protein assay despite its being only a relative method , subject to interference from Tris buffer, EDTA, nonionic and cationic detergents, carbohydrate, lipids and some salts. The incubation time is very critical for a reproducible assay. The reaction is also dependent on pH and a working range of pH 9 to 10.5 is essential.

Reagents Required

1. BSA stock solution (1mg/ml)
2. Analytical reagents:

(a) 50 ml of 2% sodium carbonate mixed with 50 ml of 0.1 N NaOH solution (0.4 gm in 100 ml distilled water.)

(b) 10 ml of 1.56% copper sulphate solution mixed with 10 ml of 2.37% sodium potassium tartarate solution. Prepare analytical reagents by mixing 2 ml of (b) with 100 ml of (a)

3. Folin-Ciocalteau reagent solution (1 N) Dilute commercial reagent (2 N) with an equal volume of water on the day of use (2 ml of commercial reagent + 2 ml distilled water)

Procedure

1. Different dilutions of BSA solutions are prepared by mixing stock BSA solution (1 mg/ ml) and water in the test tube as given in the table. The final volume in each of the test tubes is 5 ml. The BSA range is 0.05 to 1 mg/ ml.

2. From these different dilutions, pipette out 0.2 ml protein solution to different test tubes and add 2 ml of alkaline copper sulphate reagent (analytical reagent). Mix the solutions well.

3. This solution is incubated at room temperature for 10 mins.

4. Then add 0.2 ml of reagent Folin Ciocalteau solution (reagent solutions) to each tube and incubate for 30 min. Zero the colorimeter with blank and take the optical density (measure the absorbance) at 660 nm.

5. Record the absorbance in the given table.

BSA (ml)	Water (ml)	Sample conc. (mg/ml)	Sample vol. (ml)	Alk. CuSO$_4$ (ml)	Lowry reagent (ml)	O.D. 600 nm
0.25	4.75	0.06	0.2	2	0.2	
0.5	4.5	0.1	0.2	2	0.2	
1	4	0.2	0.2	2	0.2	
2	3	0.4	0.2	2	0.2	
3	2	0.6	0.2	2	0.2	
4	1	0.8	0.2	2	0.2	
5	0	1.0	0.2	2	0.2	

5. Plot the absorbance against protein concentration to get a standard calibration curve.

6. Check the absorbance of unknown sample and determine the concentration of the unknown sample using the standard curve plotted above.

Enzymes

Contents

Determination of Optimum Temperature for the Activity of Enzyme, Catechol Oxidase

Enzymes act as catalysts for the chemical reactions that occur in living organisms, allowing reactions to occur in the milliseconds necessary to maintain life.

Chemically, enzymes are proteins. Each specific enzyme has a unique physical structure that is essential for its function. The shape of each specific enzyme "fits" the shape of the reacting molecule(s) for which the enzyme serves as a catalyst. Because of the enzyme "fit", the reacting molecules are brought together at the appropriate bonding sites. The enzyme, therefore, "lowers" the activation energy of the chemical reaction.

In a reaction catalyzed by an enzyme, the reacting molecules are called the **substrate**. The substrate molecules combine with the active site of the enzyme forming a temporary complex called the **enzyme-substrate complex**. As the chemical reaction takes place and the **products** are formed, the enzyme is released, unchanged from its original structure. Since the enzyme is not consumed or changed by the chemical reaction, it can be used over and over to catalyze additional substrate molecules.

Determination of optimum temperature for the activity of enzyme, Catechol Oxidase

Catechol oxidase catalyzes the conversion of the chemical catechol to a brown pigmented substance, benzoquinone. Catechol oxidase is found in the cells of many organisms. You have probably observed this reaction a number of times when you have cut potatoes or many fruits and left them out on the counter. They turn a rusty or brownish color. The potato is a good source for this enzyme.

$$\text{Catechol} + 1/2\ O_2 \xrightarrow{\text{Catechol oxidase}} \text{1,2--Benzoquinone} + H_2O$$

71

Since catechol is colorless and the product, benzoquinone, is a rusty-brown color, the chemical reaction is easy to detect. In addition, the intensity of the pigment produced is a reflection of the amount of catechol that is converted. This, in turn, can tell you how effectively the catalyst, catechol oxidase, has worked under a set of experimental conditions.

Preparation of the Catechol Oxidase Extract (This will be done in advance by the lab staff, your instructor or by student volunteers) :

- Peel and chunk the potatoes. Put the peeled, chunked potatoes in a blender. Add 700 ml of cold distilled water and blend at high speed for 2 minutes.
- Line a large funnel with several layers of cheesecloth and place the funnel in a 1000 ml beaker, which has been placed in a container of ice. Filter the potato juice through the beaker
- The filtrate is the potato juice-catechol oxidase extract. It is called "catechol oxidase" through out the exercises.

Potatoes also contain catechol, so you will need to keep the catechol oxidase extract on ice at all times to retard any natural chemical reaction that might occur.

Standardization of the Spectrophotometer

1. Review the procedure for operating the spectrophotometer from the Spectrophotometer handout.
2. Set the wavelength to 540 nm and make any other instrument adjustments that are mentioned in the spectrophotometer handout.
3. Fill a spectrophotometer cuvette about 3/4 full of distilled water. It will be your control for the spectrophotometer.
4. Standardize the absorbance to "0" using the distilled water control cuvette.
5. Remove the blank cuvette. The spectrophotometers should have spaces to measure absorbance for four experimental cuvettes at a time.
6. Each group may have to re-standardize the spectrophotometer for the different exercises and time readings.

Cuvettes will have to be cleaned and dried after each exercise. Be sure that a cuvette that is re-used in an exercise contains the same experimental solution for each reading.

Procedure for the reference reaction

1. Label one test tube catechol oxidase and a second test tube water
2. Fill both tubes 1/4 full of distilled water
3. Add 40 drops of catechol to each tube
4. Add 160 drops of catechol oxidase (potato juice) to the catechol oxidase tube only
5. Agitate both test tubes
6. After 5 minutes, shake both tubes again and observe the results.

- The intensity of the pigment in the catechol oxidase tube will be your reference standard for the maximum reaction. You will call this intensity a "5"
- The intensity of the pigmentation (colorless) in the water tube will be your control. This intensity will be a "0".

The Effect of Temperature on Enzymatic Activity

Within limits, the rate of a chemical reaction mediated by an enzyme increases as the temperature increases. However, enzymes are proteins subject to denaturation. The maximum enzyme activity occurs at the temperature just below the point where the enzyme is denatured. Once denatured, enzyme activity rapidly declines.

In this exercise you will determine the effect of temperature on the activity of catechol oxidase at 5 different temperatures: ice water, room temperature, 40°C, 60°C and 100°C.

Setting up the experimental temperature conditions

1. There are two hot water bathes set up in the room: one at 40°C and one at 60°C
2. Set up a boiling water bath using a 600-ml beaker and a hot plate **on the side counter** for your 100°C. When the water boils, turn the hot plate down to a "simmer".
3. Fill a 600-ml beaker with crushed ice. Add water. The ice water will be about 5°C.
4. Fill a 600-ml beaker with room temperature water (about 20 –25°C).

Procedure

1. Label 5 test tubes 1 through 5.
2. Fill each tube 1/4 full of distilled water
3. Add 10 drops of catechol oxidase (potato juice) to each test tube.
4. Put Tube 1 in the ice water.

   Put Tube 2 in the beaker of room temperature water.

   Put Tube 3 in the 40°C hot water bath.

   Put Tube 4 in the 60°C hot water bath.

   Put Tube 5 in the boiling water.
5. Incubate the tubes at the designated temperatures for 10 minutes. This is to bring the tubes to the appropriate temperature. *Do not collect any data yet.*
6. After incubating the tubes for 10 minutes, add 10 drops of catechol to each of the test tube. Shake each tube vigorously.
7. Transfer contents from each of the 5 test tubes into 5 spectrophotometer cuvettes, filling each cuvette about 3/4 full. Immediately take the time "0" absorption readings for each temperature and record them in the table below. Pour the contents of each cuvette back into the appropriate test tube, shake each test tube thoroughly and return the test tubes to their

respective experimental conditions. Step 7 should be done as rapidly as possible to minimize the time the tubes are out of their experimental condition.

8. Continue to incubate the tubes at the designated temperatures. After 5 minutes shake each tube. Repeat step 7 at 5-minute intervals for a total of 10 minutes.

Enzyme Activity at different temperatures

Time (min)	Ice water	Room temp.	40°C	60°C	100°C
	Tube 1	Tube 2	Tube 3	Tube 4	Tube 5
0					
5					
10					

Plot the data for just the 10-minute interval time readings of the effect of temperature on the activity of catechol oxidase on the following graph and observe optimum temperature.

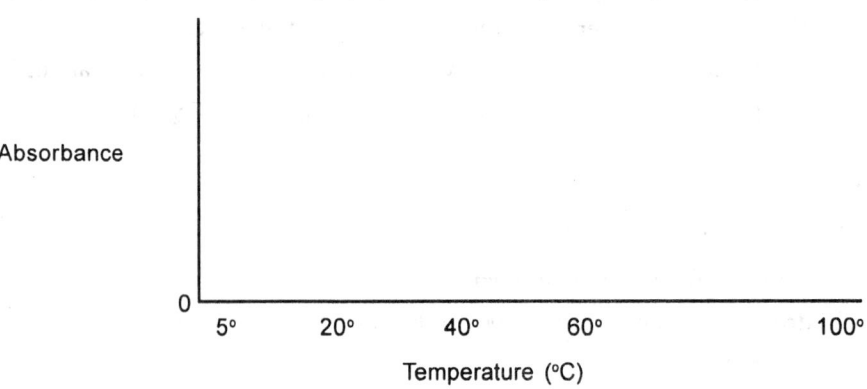

Effect of temperature on enzyme activity

Alkaloids

Contents

Introduction to Alkaloids

The earliest studies on vegetable alkalies (later termed alkaloids) date back to 1817 with German Chemist, **Sertirner** isolation of morphine. Most of the alkaloids have been discovered by Pharmacists who have obviously been interested in them for their physiological activity. Some alkaloids come from the cryptogams (non flowering plants) but most are from phanerogams.

Some unifying properties that distinguish the alkaloids include:

1. They contain nitrogen, in addition to carbon and hydrogen.
2. They are usually nonvolatile when solid but volatile when liquid.
3. They unite with aids to form ammonium salts, and theefore they are precipitated by bases.
4. Most are physiologically active, some are poisonous.
5. They are mainly crystallizable, but some are amorphous.
6. Most are white in color except berberine and sanguarnaria salts.
7. They exhibit optical activity.
8. Most are insoluble in water but soluble in organic solvents
9. Most are precipitated by Meyer,s, Marme,s, Dragendorff,s, wagner,s, Sonnenschein,s, and Schreibler,s reagents as well as gold chloride, tannic acid, and picric acid.

Alkaloidal Classification

The alkaloids are generally classified by their molecular structure and fall into 11 major caregories: pyridine-piperidine, tropane, quinoline, isoquinoline, indole, imidazole, steroidal, lupinane, alkaloidal amines, purine, plus a miscellaneous group.

1. Pyridine-piperidine class have either pyridine or piperidine and include arecoline from the betal nut, conium from the hemlock, piperine from black piper, nicotine from tobacco, and lobeline from jimson weed. Dragendorff's reagent yields a reddish-brown and bromine water gives a ycllow spot.

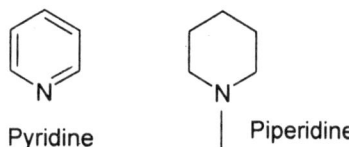

Pyridine   Piperidine

2. Tropane class have tropane structure and include atropine, cocaine, etc from aconite, hyoscyamus and stramonium. A 1% solution of cocaine yields a buff-colored spot with a $PtCl_5$ solution.

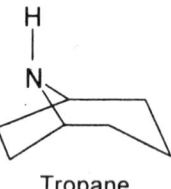

Tropane

3. Quinoline class possess a quinoline structure and include quinine obtained from cinchona bark. A 1% solution of quinine added to bromine and ammonia yields an emerald green color. A 1% solution of quinine with $AgNO_3$ yields a red to white precipitate distinct from other alkaloids.

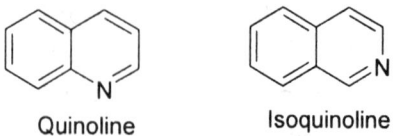

Quinoline   Isoquinoline

4. Isoquinoline class possess isoquinoline structure and include emetine from ipecac; papaverine from opium, and sanguinaria from the blood root. A sanguinaria solution in the presence of 5ml of H_2SO_4 and a drop of $FeCl_3$ yields a blue color which upon addition of HNO_3 turns to dark red-brown.

5. Indole class possess a indole structure and include strychnine from the nux vomica plant, reserpine from the rauwolfia plus physostigmine and ergot. When H_2SO_4 and 1% solution of NH_4VO_4 are added to a strychnine solution the color changes from violet to blue to purple to red. With 1.0ml of H_2SO_4 and K_2CrO_7, a deep color appears that gradually changes to violet, to cherry red, to prange and ending in yellow.

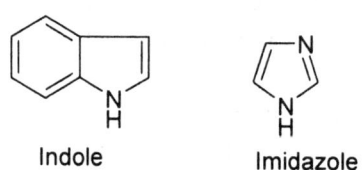

Indole   Imidazole

7. Imidazole class, containing this basic structure, includes pilocarpine from the plant *Pilocarpus jaborandi*. Pilocarpine yields a red color when treated with a solution of sodium

nitroprusside and sodium hydroxide, which on addition of sodium thiosulphate, turns green. With $K_4Fe(CN)_6$ a yellow color is produced when eventually turns to blue. A mixture of NH_4VO_4 and H_2SO_4 produces a sequence of colors from yellow to green and finally blue.

8. Steroidal class which has a basic steroid nucleus, is also known as a cyclopentenophenanthrene system. This class includes the veratrum alkaloids, as well as aconite. A solution of aconite to which is added CH_3COOH plus $KMnO_4$ yiels a red crystalline precipitate with H_3PO_4, a violet color is produced, and with HVO_4 an orange color results.

Steroid nucleus

9. Lupinine class have a undermentioned basic structure of which sparteine is an example. When sparteine is mixed with either CaI_2, phosphotungstic acid or Meyer,s reagent, a white precipitate results. With PCl_5 there is yellow precipitate, and with copper salts, a green color occurs.

Lupinine sk̇elton

10. Alkaloidal amines class have an aliphatic base plus an aromatic nucleus such as the structure of ephedrine. Colchicine also belongs to this class. Colchicine, with a couple of drops of concentrated H_2SO_4 produces a lemon yellow color. When added is added to this, the color sequence moves from greenish-blue to violet to red to yellow to colorless. With $FeCl_3$, an alcoholic solution of colchicines turns garnet red.

11. Purine class all begin with a purine system and include caffeine, theophylline, and theobromine. 50mg of theobromine heated with 1ml of $AgNO_3$ solution(10%) and 6ml of 10% NaOH solution yields a brown gelatinous mass that cannot be poured fromm the vessel.

30

Color Spot Tests for Detection of Alkaloids

Some of the major alkaloidal test solutions are:

Wagner's reagent : 2 gm of iodine and 6 gm of KI in 100 ml of water.

Meyer's reagent : 1.358 gm of $HgCl_2$ and 5 gm of KI in 100 ml of water.

Dragendorf's reagent : Potassium iodide with bismuth iodide.

Marme's reagent : 2 gm of CdI_2 and 4gm of KI in 15 ml of water.

Schreibler,s reagent : 10% solution of phosphotungstic acid.

Erdmann's reagent : 10 drops of HNO_3 in 20 ml of concentrated H_2SO_4.

Froehde's reagent : 1 gm of NH_4MoO_4 in 100 ml of H_2SO_4.

Mandelin's reagent : 1 gm of NH_4VO_4 in 200gm of H_2SO_4.

Ferric chloride solution : 8.2 gm of $FeCl_3$ in 100 ml of water.

Tannic acid solution : 1 gm of tannic acid in 100 ml of water.

Picric acid solution : 1 gm of picric acid in 100 ml of water.

0.1N iodine : 14 gm of I and 36 gm of KI in 1000 ml of water.

Experiments in Chromogenic Analysis

Color tests are widely employed for various medicinal substances. Many of these tests were serve to characterize a drug by the color of solution or precipitate formed when the drug is brought into contact with above suitable reagent. The color reagents function in a variety of ways:-

Some, such as sulphuric acid (in Froehde's and Mandelin's reagents), are powerful dehydrating agents. Other, like nitric acid, are strong oxidizers, while other rely on special reactions, such as use of ferric chloride for phenolic alkaloids.

Tannic acid, which precipitates most alkaloids, as well as some other similar substances, as white or yellowish, flocculent compounds. They are often soluble in excess of the precipitant or in other acids.

Picric acid, which from not too dilute solutions precipitates yellow compounds, often crystalline in form.

Phosphomolybdic acid precipitates the alkaloids and similar nitrogenous compounds in the form of yellowish or brownish-yellow solids. These can be filtered from the solution and the alkaloid set free from them by the alkalis and. their carbonates. *Phosphotungstic acid* acts like the phosphomolybdic in most cases.

Mercuric potassium iodide precipitates most alkaloids from solutions of their sulfuric or hydrochloric acid salts as white or yellow compounds.

Iodine in potassium iodide forms brown precipitates with alkaloidal solutions.

The following reactions are carried out by placing a few mg of the alkaloid in the depression of a white spot plate and applying the reagent with a glass rod or dropper. It is important that each reaction be observed for several minutes, since the colors formed may be transit or change rapidly through several successive shades.

Line up spot plates in the following sequence. Test reagents with blanks are listed below each spot. Record reactions, including any transient color change in each case.

Atropine
(Tropane)

H_2SO_4—
Edmann,s—
Froehde,s—
Madelin,s—
$FeCl_3$—

Sparteine
(Lupinane)

H_2SO_4—
Edmann,s—
Froehde,s—
Madelin,s—
$FeCl_3$—

Quinine
(quinoline)

H_2SO_4—
Edmann,s—
Froehde,s—
Madelin,s—
$FeCl_3$—

Strychnine
(Indole)

H_2SO_4—
Edmann,s—
Froehde,s—
Madelin,s—
$FeCl_3$—

Pilocarpine
(imidazole)

H_2SO_4—
Edmann,s—
Froehde,s—
Madelin,s—
$FeCl_3$—

Ephedrine
(Alk. Amine)

H_2SO_4—
Edmann,s—
Froehde,s—
Madelin,s—
$FeCl_3$—

Test for presence of Ergot in Food Grains

Reagents

    (a) Petroleum ether – 40–60ºC

    (b) Solvent ether

    (c) Dilute Ammonia 10% (v/v)

    (d) Tartaric acid solution – 1% (freshly prepared)

    (e) p-dimethyl amino benzaldehyde (PDAB) – Dissolve 0.125 gm of PDAB in a cold mixture of 65 ml of conc Sulphuric acid and 35 ml of distilled water. Add 0.1 ml of 5% Ferric chloride solution and let it stand for 24 hours before use.

Apparatus

    (a) Grinding mill

    (b) Electric shaker

Procedure

    (i) Grind about 50 gm of sample in the grinding mill to a fine powder. Take 10 gm of powdered sample in a stoppered conical flask.

    (ii) Add sufficient petroleum ether and shake for half an hour in the electric shaker.

    (iii) Allow to settle and decant off the petroleum ether.

    (iv) Dry the material in air. Add to the material 8 ml of dilute ammonia and sufficient quantity of solvent ether. Again shake for 30 minutes.

    (v) Filter ether portion in a beaker and concentrate to a small volume.

    (vi) Add 2 ml of tartaric acid solution to the beaker and shake thoroughly .Mix 1 ml of this tartaric acid – sample solution with 1 or 2 ml of p-dimethyl benzaldehyde solution.

    (vii) The appearance of blue color indicates presence of Ergot.

32

The Chromatography of Alkaloids

This experiment will use the principles of paper chromatography to identify a series of unknown alkaloids using known R_f factors as a guide. Paper chromatography involves the separation of substances that partition themselves a liquid stationary phase and a liquid mobile phase. To accomplish this, cut a strip of filter paper according to the width of a 1000 ml beaker. About 1 inch from the bottom of the paper, take a ruler and draw a very light pencil line parallel to the bottom of the paper. Now fill the bottom of the chromatographic chamber with the solvent mixture called for in the particular experiment. Prior to placing the filter paper down into the solvent, dissolve a few mg of six different alkaloids in a couple ml of ether, and using a small pipet or capillary tube place a drop of each dissolved alkaloid along the pencil line, spacing them proportionately. Once you have completed this operation, dry the spots over a warm heater and place the filter paper down into the solvent, making sure the level of the solvent is below the line of test spots. Place a lid on the top of the chromatographic chamber to create a vapor-tight chamber and wait for the solvents to ascend up the paper carrying the test spots to various height on the paper. When the solvents is about an inch away from the top of the paper, remove from the chamber and allow the paper to dry. For best results with alkaloids, the filter paper should be soaked in a 5% solution of sodium hydrogen citrate and dried at 60°C for 25 minutes. The solvent system used for developing the chromatogram usually consists of

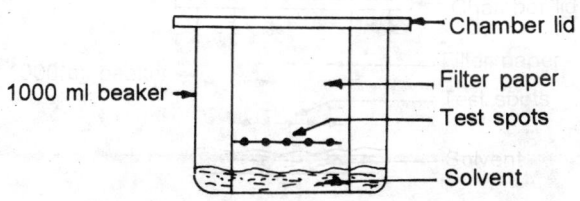

Fig. 32.1. Chromatography of alkaloids

50 ml *butanol*, 50 ml *water* and 1gm of *citric acid*. When the paper is dipped into dragendorff's reagent (5 ml each of solution A and B) plus 20 ml of acetic acid and sufficient water to make 100 ml, the alkaloids appear on the chromatogram as red spots on an orange background.

Once the chromatogram has dried you are in a position to measure the total distance moved by your solvent front(denominator in the fraction). Compare this figure with the distance moved by each of the dissolved alkaloid samples(solute). This gives you the retention factor, usually written as R_f, for each sample:

$$R_f = \frac{\text{Distance travelled by the solute}}{\text{Distance travelled by the solver}}$$

The six alkaloids for this experiment are nicotine, brucine, strychnine, atropine, physostigmine, and papaverine. Complete the column for the R_f values and compare with the values given at the end of this section. This will provide you with a partial evaluation of your accuracy in laboratory procedures. Compare results in columns 3 and 4.

Spot number	Alkaloid name	R_f value	Experimental value
1.	Nicotine	–	–
2.	Brucine	–	–
3.	Strychnine		
4.	Atropine		
5.	Physostigmine		
6.	Papaverine		

Chromatographic analysis for unknown alkaloids

In this experiment, you will follow exactly the same procedure as for the previous one, except you will be given six unknown alkaloids whose alkaloids is maintained by your lab instructor. Develop a chromatogram as before and calculate values placing them in the following table.

Alkaloid number	R_f value	Possible name of alkaloid
1.	–	–
2.	–	–
3.		
4.		
5.		
6.		

Research and replication of result over the years has led us to be able to establish some fairly well tuned R_f values for the alkaloid. Using the information from the table below, you may be able to check out the degree of accuracy of your calculation in the first experiment of this section and make a guess as to identify of the six unknowns in the second.

R_f values for Some selected alkaloids

Nicotine	0.07	Cocaine	0.39
Pilocarpine	0.11	Atropine	0.42
Morphine	0.12	Physostimine	0.47
Brucine	0.14	Papaverine	0.48
Codeine	0.16	Yohimbine	0.49
Strychnine	0.25	Veratrum	0.82

33

The Chemistry and Isolation of Hydrastine from Goldenseal

Hydrastine is a dark yellow to moderate greenish yellow powder with a distinctive odor and bitter taste and a melting point of 132ºC. It is freely soluble in acetone and benzene, but insoluble in water. It belongs to the isoquinoline class. Its structure is:-

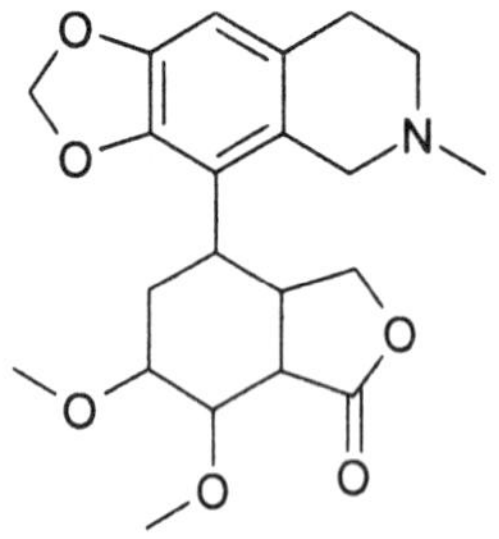

Hydrastine is claimed to be an abortifacient, antibiotic, antitussive, antiuterotic, antivaginitic, bactericide, central nervous system depressant, choleretic, convulsant, hemostat, hypertensive, hypotensive, pesticide, sedative, uterotonic, and vasoconstrictor. In the treatment of diarrhea, it has been found to have anti-microbial, antimotility, and antisecretory properties.

Experimental procedure

(i) Moist 10 gm of goldenseal (roots of *Hydrastis Canadensis*) with sufficient alkaline mixture (ammonia water, ethyl alcohol, ad ethyl ether, 1:1:8) to become damp.

(ii) Allow the moistened drug to stand in a covered container for 45 minutes.

(iii) Transfer the material to an extraction apparatus and extract the drug with ether in a soxhlet apparatus for at least 6 hours. Following this, transfer the ethereal extract to sepratory funnel and shake with three successive portion of 5% aqueous HCl.

(iv) Evaporate several ml of the extracted ether layer, dissolve the residue in a 10 ml of 5% aqueous HCl and test it with Mayer's reagent(mercuric-potassium iodide). If more faint precipitates is formed, alkaloids remain in the ether, and so the acid extraction should be repeated a fourth time.

(v) The next step is to combine the acid extracts. Make the solution alkaline to litmus with stronger ammonia water and shake it with several several portions of ether. Then check 1ml of the aqueous layer with Meyer's reagent for completeness of extraction.

(vi) Place the ether extracts in a beaker or flask and remove any water present by filtering through 20 gm of anhydrous sodium sulphate.

(vii) Place the ether extract in an evaporating disk and evaporate on a steam bath. Viii) Recrystallise the alkaloid in small beaker from hot methanol; cool with ice and scrach if necessary.

Dry the crystal on filter paper and weigh : ————

Determine the melting point point of the crystal : ————

Some color reactions of hydrastine may be illustrated by using the following procedures :

- Place a few crystals of hydrastine in a spot plate and add few drops of H_2O_2 and H_2SO_4.
  Result:————

- Place a few crystals of hydrastine in a spot plate and add few drops of H_2SO_4.
  Result:————

- Place a few crystals of hydrastine in a test tube containing 5ml of H_2SO_4.
  Result:————

"Concentrated sulphuric acid produces a yellow color, which, in contact with a crystal of potassium bichromate, becomes brown. Concentrated sulphuric acid, on warming, produces a bright red color. Concentrated nitric acid produces, in the cold, a yellow color, changing to reddish-yellow.

The Chemistry and Isolation of Berberine

Berberine is a plant alkaloid isolated from the roots and bark of several herbs. Some of these herbs include:-

Barberry (Berberis vulgaris). Berbamine and berberine are found in the plant barberry.

Coptis chinensis or Berberis aristata

Goldenseal (Hydrastis canadensis)

Oregon Grape (Berberis aquifolium)

Phellodendron Amurense

Yerba mansa (Anemopsis californica).

It is also a isoquinoline type of alkaloid which has following structure:-.

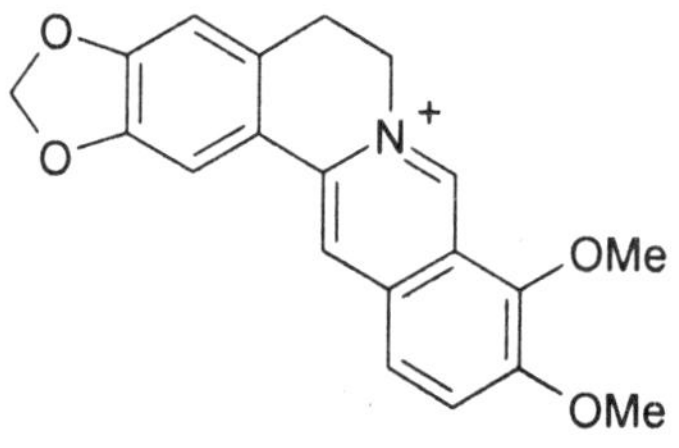

It is indicated for the treatment of fungal infection caused by **Candida albicans.**

Experimental procedure

(i) Powder the drug. Now moisten the powdered drug with ethanol, pack in column of soxhlet apparatus and extract with alcohol for 5 hrs.

(ii) Place your alcoholic extract in a beaker and evaporate over a hot plate until near dryness.

(iii) Add 50 ml of H_2O to the residue and boil to dissolve the berberine.

(iv) Filter the solution while it still hot through cotton placed in a funnel. Add 5ml of 5% HCl until the solution is acidic and allow the solution to cool.

(v) Berberine HCl will settle as dark crystal. Filter off the crystals, dry, and weigh.

Weight of berberine : ———

Determine the melting point point of the crystal : ——

Some color reactions of berberine may be illustrated by using the following procedures:

- Place a few crystals of berberine in a spot plate and add few drops of HNO_3.

  Result:————

- Place a few crystals of berberine in a test tube containing 5ml of H_2SO_4, and heat.

  Result:————

To a few crystals add a few drops of sulphuric acid and a drop of formaldehyde; yellow colour appears which changes to green.

(Note difference in reaction between hydrastine and berberine)

The Chemistry and Isolation of Nicotine from Tobbaco leaves

Nicotine is an alkoloid (a substance with a basic charge),present in the leaves of several species of plants. The primary commercial source of nicotine is by extraction from the dried leaves of tobacco plant (*Nicotinia tabaum and N. rustica*).

The chemical formula for nicotine is $C_{10}H_{14}N_2$, with a molecular mass of 162.23. In proper nomenclature, nicotine is 3-(1-Methyl-2-pyrrolidinyl) pyridine. Nicotine's structure was deduced by Pinner.The structure of nicotine is:

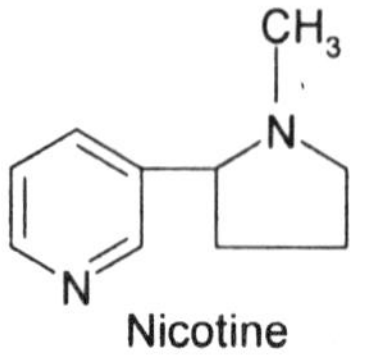

Nicotine

Isolation procedure

(i) Moisten about 50 gm of powdered drug with sufficient quantity of 20% alc. KOH solution to liberate alkaloidal base. Dry it at below 60°C.

(ii) Place the powder in flask containing 100ml of solvent ether and heat on water bath under refluxing condition for 10 minutes.

(iii) Filter and concentrate the filtrate to one fourth volume.

(iv) Treat the ethereal extract with 20 ml of dilute sulphuric acid twice.

(v) To the aqueous layer, add sufficient quantity of 5% NaOH solution.

(vi) Extract free base with solvent ether twice. Concentrate ethereal extract and dissolve in about 5ml of water and filter.

(vii) To the filtrate, add picric acid dropwise till complete precipitation of nicotine picrate take place.

(viii) Keep the solution in cold condition for 15 minutes.

(ix) Dry the product, weigh and determine its m.p.

Nicotine is isolated from tobacco by a variety of methods. Some of the most recent include supercritical CO_2 extraction, where carbon dioxide is compressed to a supercritical state (between a liquid and a gas) under high pressure, thus becoming a non-polar solvent. When the extraction is done, the CO_2 evaporates leaving behind nicotine.

Determination of Nicotine in Tobacco: A Non-Aqueous Acid-base Titration

The theory applied to acid-base titrations can also be applied to non-aqueous acid-base systems. For example, cigarettes contain several organic bases known as alkaloids? Nicotine is the most well known and abundant of these alkaloids and it has a molecular weight of 162.12 g/mol. In fact 90% of the alkaloid content in cigarettes is from nicotine or nornicotine.

In water the basicity of nicotine is too weak to permit an accurate acid-base titration. However, in an acidic non-aqueous solvent such as acetic acid, nicotine is readily quantitated by an acid base titration according to the following equation:

Experimental

(i) Into an Erlenmeyer flask accurately weigh a 6 gm sample of tobacco (6-9 cigarettes without the paper and filter components). Record this data in your lab notebook as well as the brand name of the cigarettes.

(ii) To the flasks add approximately 50 ml of the saturated aqueous $Ba(OH)_2$ solution and 2 gm of granular $Ba(OH)_2$. Insure that the tobacco is thoroughly wetted. Into the flask, pipet 100.00 ml of toluene, add a stirring bar, stopper the flask, and magnetically stir for 20 minutes.

(iii) After 20 minutes filter most of the organic layer through a whatman No.2v folded filter paper into another clean, DRY Erlenmeyer flask. The aqueous layer should not be poured into the filter.

(iv) Into a clean, DRY Erlenmeyer flask pipet 20.00 ml of the filtered solution. Add 4-5 drops of crystal violet indicator. Using your burette filled with your standardized 0.1M $HClO_4$ titrate to the characteristic greenish yellow endpoint. Repeat Step 4 two more times for reproducibility.

Factor : Each ml of 0.1 M $HClO_4$ = 0.0162 gm of nicotine.

Note : The perchloric acid is standardized by titration against potassium hydrogen phthalate.

The Chemistry and Isolation of Solasodine from Solanum SPS

It is glycoalkaloid $C_{27}H_{43}NO_2$ from plants of the Solanaceae family. It has molecular Weight: 413.3 and melting Point: 200-202°C. It is present in the berries of *Solanum khasianum* and *S.xanthocarpum* (Family Solanaccae). It is used in the partial synthesis of corticosteroids.

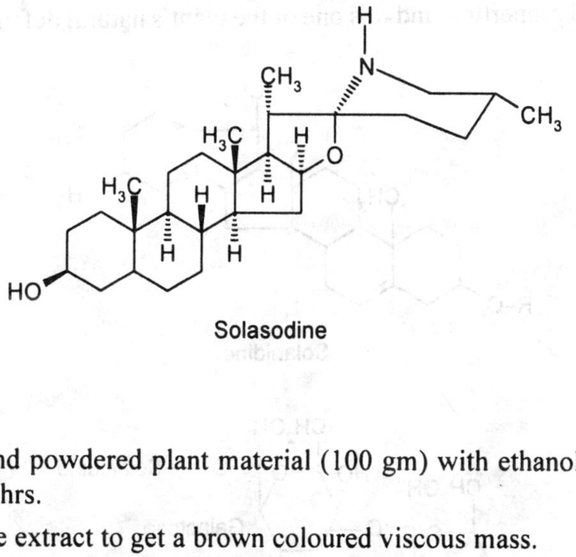

Solasodine

Isolation Procedure

(i) Extract dried and powdered plant material (100 gm) with ethanol (500 ml) in a Soxhlet apparatus for 8 hrs.

(ii) Concentrate the extract to get a brown coloured viscous mass.

(iii) Add concentrated hydrochloric acid (10 ml) and reflux the mixture for 4 hrs.

(iv) Cool down the reaction mixture below 5°C for 6 hrs and filter.

(v) To the precipitate, add few ml of hot water and adjust pH 9 with ammonia solution.

(vi) Reflux the reaction mixture for 2 hrs, cool, filter the precipitate and dry to yield about 4% of crude solasodine.

Experiment 38

The Chemistry and Isolation of Solanine from Potato

Solanine is a glycoalkaloid poison with melting point of 185°C. It can occur naturally in any part of the plant, including the leaves, fruit, and tubers. This glycoalkaloid is has a sugar component attached to a steriod-like part, solanidine. Solandine alone is much less toxic. The sugar is necessary for the extreme toxicity. Solanine is very poisonous even in very small quantities. Hence, Solanine has both fungicidal and pesticidal properties, and it is one of the plant's natural defenses.

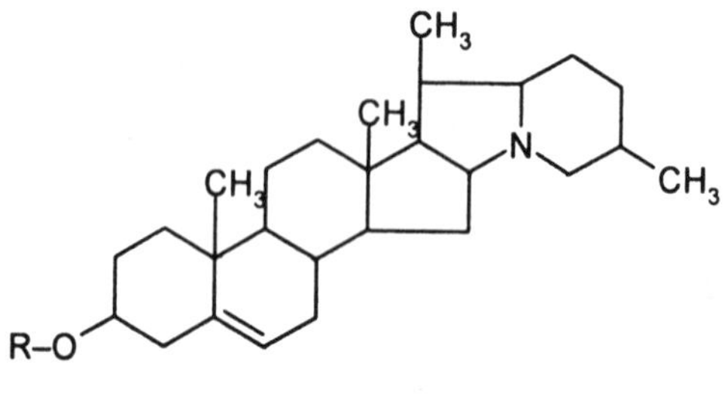

Solanidine

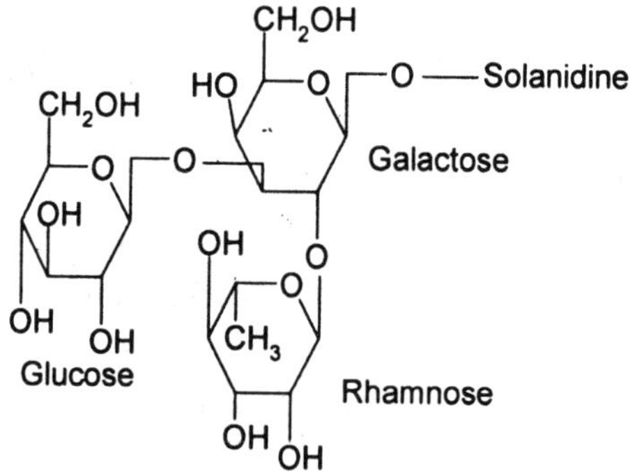

Solanine

Solanine occurs naturally in all nightshades, including tomatoes, capsicum, tobacco and eggplant, as well as plants from other species. However the most ingested solanine is from the consumption of potatoes.

Isolation Procedure

(i) Macerate the pieces of potatoes (500 gm) with 5% acetic acid (2 litre) for 24 hrs.

(ii) Warm to 70°C, cool and adjust pH to 9.5 with ammonia solution.

(iii) Centrifuge, wash the precipitate with sufficient amount of 1% ammonia solution and centrifuge again.

(iv) Discard the supernatant liquid and washing.

(v) Dry and weigh the residue.

(vi) Purify it by dissolving in boiling methanol, filtering and concentrating until the glycoalkaloid starts to crystallize.

The Chemistry and Isolation of Strychnine from Nux Vomica

The dried, ripe seeds of *Strychnos Nux-vomica* Linné (Fam. *Loganiaceae*), yielding not less than 2.5 per cent. of the alkaloids of Nux Vomica. The therapeutic value of nux vomica is due entirely to the two alkaloids, brucine and strychnine, although there are other substances present of some interest. Strychnine and its relative, brucine, are both members of the indole class of alkaloids. Their structures are:

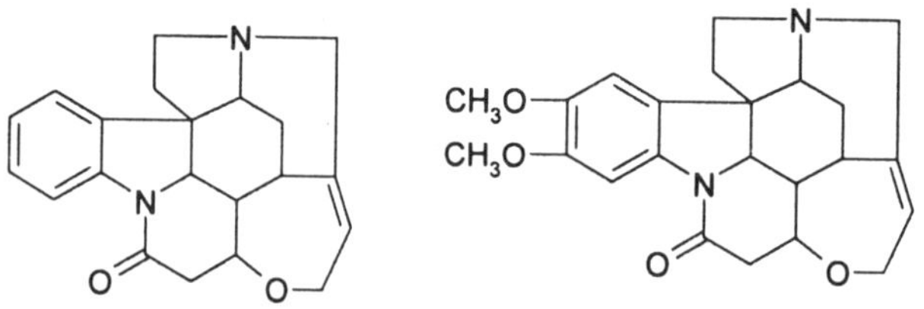

Strychnine

Brucine
(Dimethoxy strychnine)

Isolation procedure

(i) Place 10 gm of nux vomica powder being placed in a flask containing 30 ml chloroform, 50 ml of ether, and 5 ml of 10% ammonia water.

(ii) Shake the mixture frequently during 45 minutes, and the filter through cotton and transferred to a separatory funnel. Add dilute H_2SO_4 and shake well.

(iii) Take the lower aqueous layer, which should have an acid reaction when tested with litmus paper, into a second separatory funnel and the ether-chloroform extracted twice more with acid. Combine acid extracts containing the alkaloids from the original drug and make alkaline with dilute ammonia water to liberate alkaloidal base.

(iv) Extract this by shaking with several portions of chloroform.

(v) After the chloroform extractions are washed with a little water, evaporate off the solvents by heating in an evaporating dish.

(vi) Add the little ethyl alcohol and at once evaporate off, and dry the residue, consisting of strychnine and brucine, at 100^0C and weigh.

Record the weight of the alkaloidal mixture ——————————————

(vii) The process for separating strychnine from brucine depends on the greater readiness by which brucine is nitrated with HNO_3.(*Note. The separation of brucine from strychnine is most conveniently effected by exposing the mixed alkaloids to the action of diluted nitric acid, which destroys brucine very rapidly while having no appreciable action on strychnine).*

(vii) Dissolve the alkaloidal mixture in 10ml of dilute H_2SO_4. Using 50ml of H_2O, filter into a graduated cylinder. Pour the cylinder content into a flask and add exactly 5ml of concentrated HNO_3. The addition of HNO_3 should cause the solution to attain a crimson color. After standing for exactly 15 minutes, transfer the liquid to a separatory funnel and at once make alkaline with NaOH solution, and extract the strychnine with three portions of chloroform in a usual way. After boiling off the chloroform in an evaporating dish, add a little ethyl alcohol and evaporate to dryness. After drying at 100^0C, weigh the residue of strychnine.

Note : *Brucine may be separated from strychnine by virtue of the lesser solubility of its oxalate in dehydrated alcohol or of its hydriodide in water, or by the insolubility of strychnine chromate in water. Potassium ferrocyanide precipitates the strychnine from a hydrochloric acid solution of the alkaloids, the brucine remaining in solution. Brucine is crystallizable from aqueous alcohol, the crystals then contain $4H_2O$. It is without odor, but of a permanent, harsh, very bitter taste; is sparingly soluble in water; very soluble in alcohol, whether hot or cold; it dissolves in 4 parts of chloroform, 440 parts of ether, 60 parts of benzene, and 120 parts of petroleum benzin. It is permanent in the air. The hydrated crystals melt at 105° C., while the anhydrous base melts at 178° C., changing color, and depositing carbon. It forms crystallizable salts with acids.*

Result : Color tests are available to differentiate between strychnine and brucine. Conduct the following tests and record results.

To a 0.1gm of strychnine, add 1ml of a 50:50 mixture of concentrated HNO_3 and H_2O and record result of spot test : ————

There is no appreciable action on strychnine.

Perform the same test with 0.1 gm of brucine.

Concentrated nitric acid produces with brucine or its salts an intense crimson color, which changes to yellow by heat.

Now add a few drops of the water to the brucine and add a few drops of stannous chloride.

Results : ——————————

The yellow liquid becomes violet upon the addition of stannous chloride or ammonium or sodium sulphide.

The Chemistry and Isolation of Piperine from Black Pepper

Piperine is the alkaloid responsible for the pungency of black pepper along with chavicine (an isomer of piperine). It has also been used in some forms of traditional medicine and as an insecticide.

Piperine is a solid substance essentially insoluble in water. It is a weak base that is tasteless at first, but leaves a burning after taste. Piperine belongs to the vanilloid family of compounds, a family that also includes capsaicin, the pungent substance in hot chili peppers. Piperine is the trans-trans stereoisomer of 1-piperoylpiperidine. It is also known as (*E, E*)-1-piperoylpiperidine and (*E, E*)-1-[5-(1, 3-benzodioxol-5-y1)-1-oxo-2, 4-pentdienyl] piperidine. It is represented by the following chemical structure:

Piperine

Isolation procedure

Method I : Place 15 gm of powdered black pepper in a 250 ml round-bottomed flask, add 150 ml of 95% ethanol and 5 boiling chips, and heat at reflux for 2 hrs. Filter the mixture by suction filtration and then concentrate the filtrate to a volume of 10-15 ml by simple distillation or by use of a rotary evaporator. To 10 ml of a 10% solution of KOH in 95% ethanol contained in a 125 ml erlenmeyer flask, add the concentrated pepper extract. Heat the resulting solution and add water dropwise. a yellow precipitate forms. Add water until no more solid appears to form and then allow the mixture to stand at least overnight. Collect the solid by suction filtration and recrystallize it with 10-20 ml of acetone.

(i) This extraction may be scaled up to twice the amounts specified without difficulty. If a soxhlet extractor is available, this would be an apparatus superior to a standard reflux setup.

(ii) Boiling chips are necessary to prevent serious bumping.

(iii) It is best to allow piperine to completely precipitate out by allowing the mixture to stand until the next laboratory period.

(iv) In our hands 0.6gm of piperine, mp 127-128°C, was collected upon recrystallization.

Method II : Extract the powdered black pepper(10gm) with 95% ethanol(150ml) in a soxhlet extractor for 2hrs. Filter the solution and concentrate in vacuum on a water bath at 60°C. Add 10ml 10% alcoholic KOH solution and decant after a while from the insoluble residue. Leave the alcoholic solution left overnight, where upon 0.3gm yellow needles are deposited, mp 125-126°C.

TLC of black pepper extract : The crude extract is spotted on a thin-layer plate using silica gel G as adsorbent and developed with benzene:Ethyl acetate 2:1.

Detection :

(i) UV365 shows blue fluorescence of piperine

(ii) spraying with anisaldehyde-sulphric acid reagent, prepared by mixing 0.5 ml anisaldehyde with 10ml glacial acetic acid, 85 ml MeOH, and 5mL concentrated sulphric acid. this solution is sprayed on the plate, which is then heated at 110°C for 10min. piperine appears as a yellow spot, R_f 0.25.

Method III : The piperine, a very weakly basic substance, can be isolated from a variety of peppers by extraction with alcohol. The piperine, along with a small amount of its Z, E isomer, accounts for about 10% of the weight of black pepper.

Place 15 gm of ground black pepper and 1gm of powdered $CaCO_3$ in a 250 ml boiling flask, add 100ml of Isopopyl alcohol(PA), and, after fitting the flask with a reflux condenser, boil the mixture for about 1hr on the steam bath. At the end of the heating period, filter the mixture by gravity into a 125ml erlenmeyer flask. Boil off all solvent but about 10ml of the IPA.

Transfer the residual solution from the boiling flask to a 25ml erlenmeyer flask, and set the flask aside to cool for crystallization of piperine. Collect the product by suction filtration, using small portions of MeOH to rinse the flask and wash theproduct.yield:about 0.5 gm.

(i) The addition of $CaCO_3$ should prevent the extraction of acidic components of pepper.

(ii) IPA boils at 80°C, only a little below the maximum temperature attainable on the steam bath. to make the distillation proceed quickly, clamp the boiling flask so that it is well down in the rings of the steam bath, and drape a towel over the flask and the steam bath to make a tent that will hold steam around the top of the flask.

(iii) Crystallization occurs slowly, and the flask must be allowed to stand for at least 24hrs.

(iv) Alternatively, add 25ml of water to the IPA solution of piperine, allow the mixture to stand for at least 24hrs so that precipitation will be complete, collect the solid by sucction filtration, and recrystallize it from either IPA or acetone.

Method IV : Add 5 gm of pure ground pepper and 10ml of CH_2Cl_2 to 50 ml round-bottomed flask.

Use the round-bottom flask as the basis for a reflux apparatus having water cooled-condenser and heating mantle. Heat the sample to reflux, and then maintain a gentle reflux for 20min. after the required reflux period, lower the heating mantle and allow the reflux apparatus to cool for 5min. Suction filter the slurry with the aid of a 4.5 cm buchner funnel, washing the pepper grounds once with 5ml of CH_2Cl_2. Remove 2 or 3 drops of the extract and place it in a capped vial for use in the TLC analysis.

Trituration/isolation

Transfer the extract obtained above to a clean 25 ml round-bottomed flask and concentrate in vacuo. The resulting olive-brown, viscous oil should be cooled in an ice-bath and then 3ml of cold ether added to the oil while gently stirring for 3-4 minutes. Some piperine may precipitate at this point, but remove the solvent in vacuum anyway. Once again cool the resulting oil in an ice-bath and then add 3ml of cold ether to the oil while gently stirring to promote the precipitation of piperine. Allow the flask to cool for an additional 10min with occasional stirring. Isolate the straw-yellow crystals of crude piperine by suction filtration with the aid of a 1.5cm harsch funnel. Wash the crystals twice with 2ml portions of cold ether. Place a small portion of the filtrate in a capped vial for use in the TLC analysis.

Recrystallization

Place the crude piperine isolated above into a 13 × 100 mm test tube and dissolve it in a minimum amount of hot acetone: hexane solution 3:2). Once all the solid has dissolved, allow the test tube to sit undisturbed for 15min at room temperature. Rod-like, yellow crystals of piperine should be present. Cool the solution for an additional 30 min in an ice-bath before isolating the purified piperine by suction filtration with the help of a 1.5 cm harsch funnel. Wash the crystals once with a 2 ml portion of cold ether, allow them to air dry for several minutes. Typically, yields of approximately 2% or 100 mg are obtained. The melting point of the purified piperine now can be determined and the identity of the product confirmed by mixed melting point, TLC analysis, or spectral analysis.

Hydrolysis of Piperine – Isolation of Piperic Acid

Reflux a solution of 1 gm of piperine in 10 ml of 10% alcoholic KOH for 90 minutes. Evaporate the solution to dryness by distillation under reduced pressure, the receiver being cooled in an ice-salt bath. Suspend the solid potassium piperinate remaining in the distillation flask in hot water and add concentrated HCl.

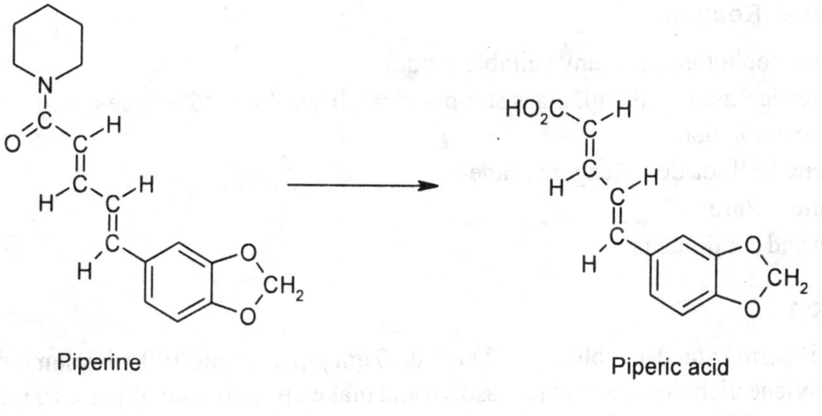

Piperine   Piperic acid

Collect the yellow precipitate, wash it with ice-cold water and recrystallise it from ethanol. Pure piperic acid is obtained as yellow needles, m.p. 216–217°C.

Determination of Piperine Content

Principle

Piperine is extracted into Ethylene dichloride ($C_2H_4Cl_2$) and UV absorptionis measured at maximum 342-345 nm The concentration is determined from a standard curve prepared with known quantities of pure piperine. Other isomers of piperine that may be present and related compounds such as piperettine and piperylin which also absorb at 340-345 will also be included.

Apparatus and Reagents

  (a) UV spectrophotometer – any suitable model
  (b) Volumetric flasks – 100 ml, glass stoppered, amber colored to reduce photo degradation of piperine in solution.
  (c) Ethylene Dichloride – Reagent grade
  (d) Piperine – Pure
  (e) Spices and condiments

Determination

Preparation of Piperine Standard solution – Weigh 0.10 gm piperine into 100 ml volumetric flask, add about 70 ml ethylene dichloride, shake to dissolve and make up to volume. Pipette 10 ml into 100 ml volumetric flask and dilute to volume. Pipette 1, 2, 3, 4, 5, 6 ml aliquots into six 100 ml volumetric flasks and dilute to volume with ethylene dichloride. Adjust to zero absorbance spectrophotometer with ethylene dichloride and read absorbance of each final solution at maximum 342-345 nm using UV light source and ethylene dichloride in reference cell. Plot a graph of concentration against observed absorbance

Procedure

  (i) Grind sample to pass 60 mesh sieve and blend uniformly. Accurately weigh 0.5 gm test sample and transfer to 125 Erlenmeyer flask. Protect from light.

(ii) Add about 70 ml ethylene dichloride. Reflux and stir 1 hour, cool to room temperature and filter quantitatively through paper into 100 ml volumetric flask. Transfer rest of the extracted residue to filter, wash thoroughly and dilute to volume.

(iii) Pipette 2 ml of this solution into 100 ml volumetric flask and dilute to volume. Record absorbance at maximum 342-345 nm Obtain percentage of piperine content from the calibration curve

Isolation of Total Vasaka Alkaloids from Vasaka leaves

The medicinal properties of *Adhatoda vasica* Nees (Natural Order: Acanthaceae), called Vasa or Vasaka in Sanskrit, have been known in India and several other countries for thousands of years. The plant has been recommended by Ayurvedic physicians for the management of various types of respiratory disorders.

The major bioactive constituent of Adhatoda vasica is a pyrralazoquinoline alkaloid – vasicine. The other alkaloids include vasicol, adhatonine, vasicinone, vasicinol, vasicinolone etc. The vasicinone is a autooxidation product of vasicine.

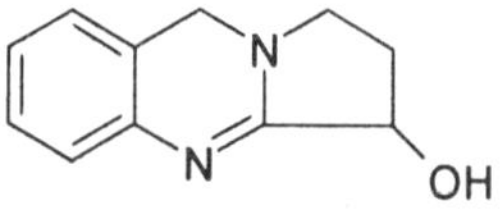

Vasicine 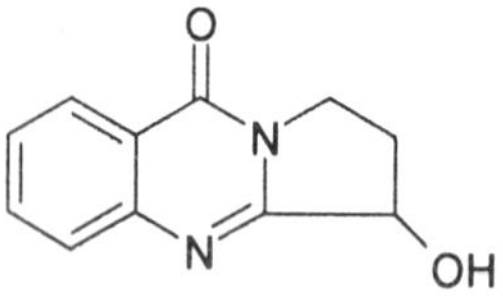   Vasicinone

Isolation procedure

1. Extract the dried and pulverized leaves(100gm) of Adhatoda vasica with 500ml of an alcohol(80%) extract at an ambient temperature by maceration process for 24 hrs with intermittent stirring.
2. Concentrate the alcoholic extract to about its one tenth volume and add 2% acetic acid(organic acid) to acidify it and allow to stand for 2hrs.
3. Extract the concentrated extract with chloroform twice, each of 50ml.
4. Separate out the acidic layer and basify it with with aqueous ammonia solution.
5. Extract the basified extract with chloroform.
6. Separate out organic layer, dry it, filter and evaporate to get amorphous residue.
7. The amorphous residue is a mixture of alkaloids but vascine may be separated by treatment/ crystallization with organic solvent or mixture of organic solvents

The Chemistry and Isolation of Quinine from Cinchona Bark

Quinine is the most important alkaloid, obtained from Cinchona bark. It belongs to quinoline group having following structure:-

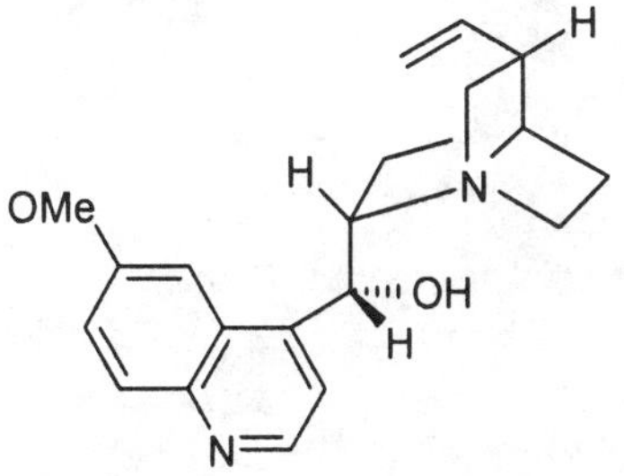

This alkaloid is colorless, amorphous, or in acicular crystals, very bitter; soluble in 1670 parts water, 6 parts alcohol, 26 parts ether. Aqueous solutions of the salts have a blue fluorescence, and when treated with chlorine water and ammonia a beautiful green color is produced—"Thalleoquin test." It has been used for many years as an antimalarial agent. Although it does not cure malaria, it is effective in alleviating the symptoms of malarial attacks. The usual medicinal form is quinine dihydrochloride or quinine sulphate dihydrate,

Isolation procedure

(i) Moisten powdered cinchona(50gm) with ammonia water and allow it to stand for an hour, then hot water is added. To the mixture, after cooling, milk of lime is added and the whole evaporated to dryness.

(ii) Dry at room temperature or below 60^0C temperature.

(iii) Pack the material in soxhlet apparatus and extract with benzene for 6 hrs.

(iv) Extract the benzene extract with dilute sulphuric acid under stirring condition.

(v) Separate the acidic aqueous liquid, neutralize the acidulated layer and allow to stand when neutral sulphates of the alkaloid (quinine, cinchonine, cinchonidine) are crystallized out.

(vi) Dissolve the crude quinine sulphate in water, decolorized with charcoal and recrystallized until the cinchonidine and cinchonine are reduced to the required percentage.

(vii) Determine its melting point(m.p.177ºC)

45

The Chemistry and Isolation of Caffeine from Tea

Caffeine ($C_8H_{10}N_4O_2$) is the common name for trimethylxanthine (systematic name is 1,3,7-trimethylxanthine or 3,7-dihydro-1,3,7-trimethyl-1H-purine-2,6-dione). The chemical is also known as coffeine, theine, mateine, guaranine, or methyltheobromine. The structure of caffeine is:

Caffeine

When purified, caffeine is an intensely bitter white powder. It is added to colas and other soft drinks to impart a pleasing bitter note. It is soluble in water, alcohol, acetone, chloroform, benzene, and ether. Solubility in water is increased by the presence of alkali, benzoates, cinnamates, citrates, or salicylates.

Caffeine is found in tea leaves, coffee beans, kola nuts, and cocoa beans. For the plants, caffeine acts as a natural pesticide. It paralyzes and kills insects that attempt to feed on the plants. The Table below gives the amount of caffeine in the various beverages prepared from these natural products.

One can develop both a tolerance and a dependence on caffeine. The dependence is real, and a heavy [> 5 cups of coffee per day] user will experience lethargy, headache, and perhaps nausea after about 18 hrs abstinence. An excessive intake of caffeine may lead to restlessness, irritability, insomnia, and muscular tremor. Caffeine can be toxic, but it has been estimated that to achieve a lethal dose of caffeine one would have to drink about 100 cups of coffee over a relatively short time.

Because of the central nervous system effects that caffeine causes, many persons prefer to use decaffeinated coffee. The caffeine is removed from coffeeby extracting the whole beans with trichloroethylene at 71°C. Following this, the solvent is drained off, and the beans are steamed to remove any residual solvent. Then, the beans are dried and roasted to bring out the flavor. Decaffeination reduces the caffeine content of coffee from a range of 2% to 5% to the range of 0.03% to 1.2% caffeine.

Table : The amount of caffeine found in beverages*

Brewed Coffee	60-100 mg/100 ml
Decaffeinated Coffee	18-35 mg/100 ml
Tea	18-53 mg/100 ml
Coca-Cola	12 mg/100 ml
Cocoa	3.5 mg/100 ml

* The average cup of coffee or tea contains about 150 ml of liquid.
The average bottle of Coke contains about 350 ml of liquid.

Isolation procedure

The isolation of caffeine from tea leaves presents the chemist with a major problem: caffeine does not occur alone in tea leaves, but is accompanied by other natural substances from which it must be separated. The major components of tea leaves are:

1. Cellulose - the major structural material of all plant cells. Since cellulose is virtually insoluble in water it presents no problems in the isolation procedure.
2. Caffeine - one of the major water soluble substances present in tea leaves. Caffeine comprises as much as 5% by weight of the leaf material in tea plants.
3. Tannins - high molecular weight, water soluble compounds that are responsible for the color of tea. The term "tannin" does not refer to a single compound or even to substances having similar chemical structure. Rather, "tannin" refers to a class of compounds that have certain properties in common. They contain phenol groups, are acidic and are used to convert animal hides to leather [tanning].
4. Flavonoid Pigments - water soluble colored compounds that are widely distributed in plant life.
5. Chlorophylls - water soluble green plant pigments that enable plants to convert carbon dioxide and water to carbohydrates and oxygen[photosynthesis].

Experimental Procedure

(i) Place 50 gm of a powdered tea and 250 ml of water in a 600 ml beaker and boil gently for 30 minutes.
(ii) Strain the resulting hot extract through muslin. Carefully add a solution of basic lead acetate $[Pb(C_2H_2O_2)_2]$ to the filtrate until no more precipitate forms.
(iii) Heat the mixture to boiling and filter through a Buchner funnel and vacuum system. Heat the filtrate to boiling and then add slowly dilute sulphuric acid until precipitation of lead sulphate occurs.

Flow diagram for the separation of caffeine from tea leaves

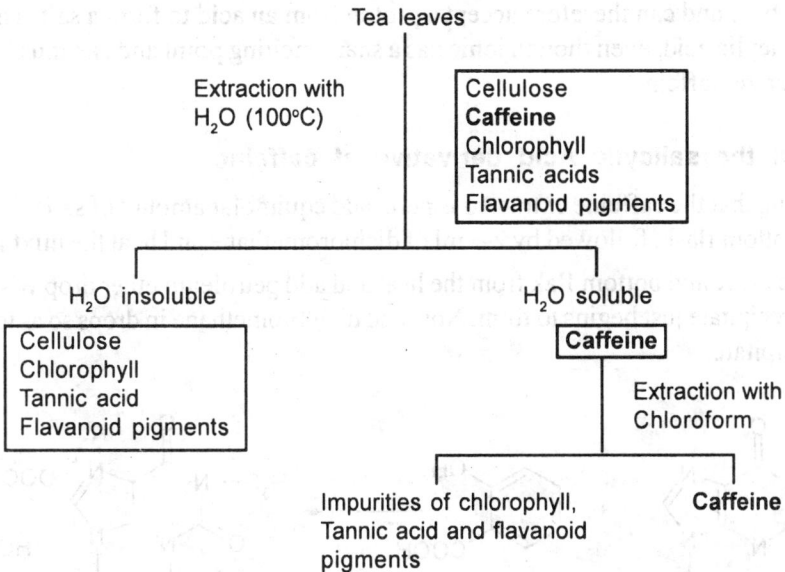

(iv) Add approximately 1 gm of decolorizing charcoal to the mixture, which is boiled for a few minutes and then filter.

(v) Cool the filtrate and transfer to a separatory funnel and shake out with three successive 10 ml portion of chloroform. Transfer the combined extracts to a small evaporating dish and warm to dryness,

(vi) Dry the combined $CHCl_3$ extracts with anhydrous sodium sulphate. Swirl for several minutes to allow enough time for the sodium sulphate to become hydrated with the water.

(vii) Filter the dry $CHCl_3$ solution into a dry pre-weighed 100 mL round-bottom flask. Wash the filter paper and drying agent with about 1ml of $CHCl_3$.

(viii) Either Remove the $CHCl_3$ by simple distillation or rotaevaporate off the solvent, until about 5 ml of liquid remains in the round-bottom flask. Do not allow the flask to go dry otherwise the caffeine may decompose.

(ix) Place the round-bottom flask on a steam bath and evaporate the contents to dryness at low-medium heat.

(x) Weigh the flask to find the crude mass of caffeine.

(xi) Scrape out the residue, transfer to a small beaker and dissolve in a small amount of hot CH_3OH. Let stand overnight and filter off the caffeine crystals.

(xii) Record weight of the caffeine.

(xiii) Determine the melting point point of the crystal : The caffeine isolated from tea leaves can be purified by sublimation. Caffeine melts and sublimes at 238ºC. But during this experiment you will identify caffeine not from its melting point but from the melting point of its salicylate.

One way to identify an organic compound is to prepare a derivative of it. Caffeine is an organic base and can therefore accept a proton from an acid to form a salt. The salt formed from salicylic acid, even though ionic has a sharp melting point and can thus be used to help characterize caffeine.

Preparation of the salicylic Acid derivative of caffeine

(i) Assuming that the caffeine extracted is pure, add equimolar amount of salicylic acid into the round bottom flask, followed by 2-3 ml of dichloromethane and heat the mixture to boiling

(ii) Remove the round bottom flak from the heat and add petroleum ether drop wise until a solid white precipitate just begins to form. Now add dichloromethane in drops so as to just dissolve the precipitate.

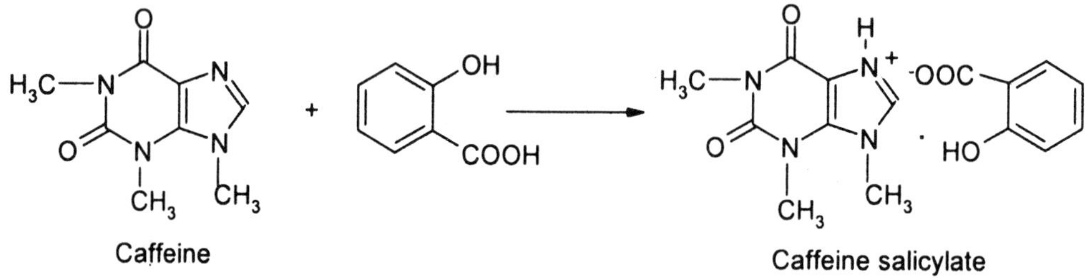

Caffeine   Caffeine salicylate

(iii) Let the solution cool very slowly to room temperature and then put it on ice to aid the crystallization.

(iv) Vacuum filter the crystals using a Hirsh funnel and rinse with pertroleum ether.

(v) Find the mass and the melting point of caffeine salicylate. Transfer the product into a vial and submit the labeled vial for marking.

Some Color Reactions of Caffeine

Some color reactions of caffeine may be illustrated by using the following procedures:

- In a watch glass, mix a small amount of your sample with 2-3 drops of concentrated hydrochloric acid. Use a glass rod for mixing. Add a few small crystals of potassium chlorate and mix well. Heat the watch glass over a boiling water bath until the sample is dry. Allow to cool. Moisten with a drop of 'bench' (2 mol dm^{-3}) ammonia solution. Observe the color change. Add few drops to NaOH solution and again observe the change in color.

   Result : —————

This test is known as Murexide color test. A strong purple-red color is produced due to formation of murexide, a violet compound. Chemically, it is ammonium purpurate. The violet color disappears on addition to NaOH solution.

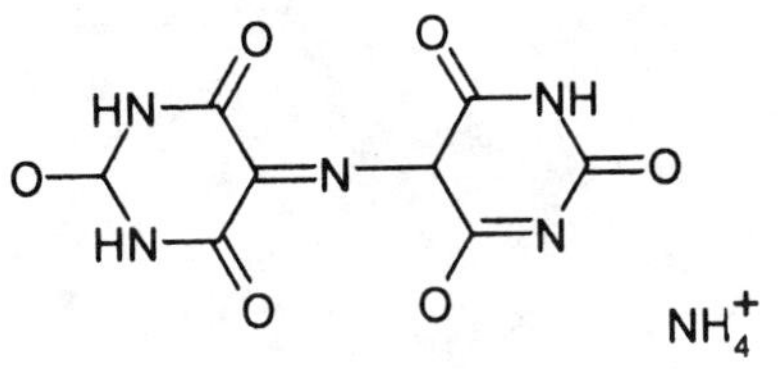

Murexide

Murexide is a useful indicator for metals complexes such as nickel. The nickel complex is yellow.

- To 5ml of a saturated solution of caffeine, add 5 drops of iodine. The add 3 drops of diluted HCl.

   Result:—————

   It should give brown precipitate.

111

- Add tannic acid to a saturated solution of caffeine.

  A white precipitate of caffeine tannate is produced.

Chromatographic procedure

1. Solvents. Mix Iso-BuOH: AcOH: H_2O (10: 1: 2.4) and shake until clear. Use this solution as the mobile phase. Take a small portion of the mobile phase and shake with water (100 ml) until it is water saturated. Draw this aqueous layer and use for equilibration of the chromatographic chamber.

2. Paper treatment. Dip Whatman 3 MM paper (18" x 22") sheets in 0.5 M aqueous potassium dihydrogen phosphate (pH 4.2) and ammonium sulphate (2%, pH 5.3), dry and use for the preparation of the chromatograms;

3. Standard drug reference solutions. Reference standards of the caffeine is prepared by dissolving the base (50 mg) in methanol (10 ml) and stored at 4°C until required. Spot the reference solution and test sample on chromatogram.

4. Run the chromatogram, dry it and spray with Modified Dragendorff Ludy-Tenger reagent. (Bismuth subcarbonate (1 gm) and potassium iodide (6 gm) and hydrochloric acid (conc., 15 ml) were diluted with water to 100 ml. The reagent at this concentration may be further diluted (1: 1) with water, if desired for respraying faded chromatograms). Caffeine yield orange spots.

UV Determination of Caffeine Content in Selected Soft Drinks

Caffeine is a common organic molecule found in many beverages such as coffee, tea, and cola. It is a stimulant to the central nervous system. That is why many students drink coffee or soda to help them feel alert.

Like many conjugated organic molecules, caffeine absorbs radiation with a wavelength around 260 nm. A conjugated system is one containing 2 double bonds separated by a single bond. This conjugated pattern may be repeated several times in the molecule. If a series of caffeine standards are analyzed in this region of absorption and a Beer's law is plot prepared, then the amount of caffeine in another substance can be determined. One should be aware that the assumption is being made that the unknown contains no other substances which absorb at this wavelength.

Procedure

1. Prepare 50.00 ml of the assigned caffeine standard (50, 100, 150, 200, or 250 ppm) by a quantitative dilution of the 1000 ppm stock solution.

2. Place the caffeine standard in a separatory funnel. Add 25 ml of methylene chloride.

3. Extract the caffeine by inverting the funnel at least 3 times. Vent the separatory funnel after each inversion.

4. Remove the methylene chloride layer, which is the bottom layer, and save in a clean, stoppered Erlenmeyer flask.

5. Add another 25 ml of methylene chloride to the separatory funnel.

6. Extract twice more by repeating steps 3-5. Combine the methylene chloride layers.

7. Add 50 ml of degassed soda to a clean separatory funnel (the separatory funnel may be rinsed with methylene chloride to be certain that no caffeine from the previous sample remains).

8. Extract the soda 3 times with 25 ml portions of methylene chloride as above. Save the methylene chloride layers in another clean, stoppered Erlenmeyer flask.

9. Fill a clean cuvet with methylene chloride. Wipe the unfrosted sides with a Kimwipe. Place the cuvette in the sample compartment in U.V spectrophotometer with the unfrosted sides facing the front and back. Close the lid.

10. Press the green button under "Collect Baseline" and wait for the collection to be completed. (The baseline will be stored in the instrument, but will not appear on the screen. "Baseline Collected" will appear when the scan is complete).

11. Remove the blank and dump the contents into a waste container. Rinse the cuvette into the waste container twice with small amounts of sample. Fill the cuvette ¾ full with sample. Return the cuvette to the sample compartment and measure the absorbance at 260nm.

12. Repeat same steps with the other standards and unknown solutions. Remember to label the printouts with the sample name.

13. Plot a Beer's law curve of absorbance (y) vs concentration (x) for the caffeine standards. From the standard curve, read out the concentration of various soft drink.

Observation Table

Caffeine standards		Soft drinks		
Concentration (ppm)	Absorbance	Brand	Concentration Absorbance (ppm)	Caffeine mg/ml
0.00				
50.00				
100.00				
150.00				
200.00				
250.00				

Calculations

1. Using the graph, determine the concentration of caffeine in each soda in ppm.
2. Calculate the mg of caffeine in a 12 oz serving (253 ml) of soft drinks.

Assay of Belladonna for Hyoscyamine Content

Alkaloidal assays are commonly performed for pupeses of standardization, proof of purity, commercial evaluation, or pharmacological purposes. A slight deficiency of alkaloid in a preparation may cause a marked decrease in physiological efet, or a slight excess may cause toxic effects when the preparation is administered.

The amount of alkaloids that occurs in crude drugs are subject to considerable variation in different samples of the same drug. The variations may be caused by:

1. The age of the plant when it is administered.
2. The season of the year when the drug is harvested.
3. The soil and climate the drug is grown
4. The conditions under when the drug is collected, stored, and dried.

In view of the fact that alkaloids may comprise only a fraction 0f 1% of the substance assayed and that this small amount must be separated from numerous other constituents present in the crude drug, such as reseins, volatile oils, coloring matter, glycosides, fatty acids, gums, and proteins, it is evident that the exact technique involved in any given method must be carefully adhered to in order to estimate the variation in alkaloidal content. It is this special technique that characterizes the chemical assay of drugs, rather than the gravimetric or volumetric nature of the procedure employed.

Alkaloidal Determination in Belladonna

Place 10 gm of belladonna powder in a dry flask and macerate with mixture of 10 ml of ethanol and 20 ml of ether for 10 minutes, then add 5ml of ammonia water to ender the solution alkaline and liberate the alkaloidal bases from their salts. Allow to stand with frequent shaking for an hour and then transfer the contents of the flask to a small percolator as shown in the diagram. Percolate the drug first with another ether-alcohol mixture and then with ether alone, until the alkaloids are extracted. In order to ascertain when complete extraction has taken place, a few drops of the solvent is collected on watch glass and the solvent evaporated. To a residue, add a drop of HCl and a couple drops of

Meyer's reagent, if the extraction is incomplete, a cream-colored precipitate or turbidity indicative of the presence of alkaloid will appear. Once the liquid remains clear, extraction is complete. Owing to the tendency of the alkaloids to hydrolyze during extraction, the percolation should not last more than three hours.

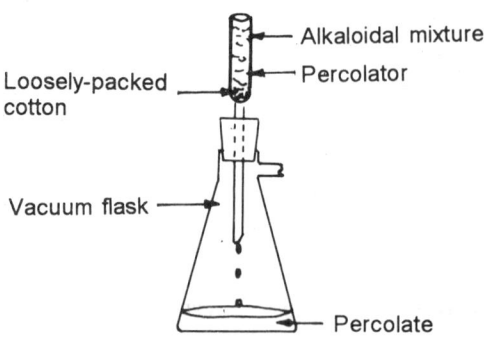

Fig. 48.1. Percolation

Transfer the percolate to a separatory funnel and shake with an excess of dilute HCl. After separation, the lower level is drawn off into another separatory funnel and the ethereal layer twice more extracted with small portions of dilute HCl mixed a little alcohol. In this way, the alkaloids are transferred from there to the aqueous acid liquid. Add the alcohol to prevent the formation of troublesome emulsions. The acid solution of the alkaloids is now freed from traces of chlorophyll and extractive matter with 10ml of chloroform, allowing to separate and drawinig off the chloroformic liquid into another separatory funnel and the shaking with a little dilute acid in order to remove any traces of alkaloids which may have passed into the chloroform.

After separation, reject the chloroform and make the acidic solution now alkaline with 10ml of ammonia water. This liberates the alkaloidal bases, which are sparingly soluble in water, and they can be extracted by shaking with several successive portion of chloroform. Evaporate off the chloroform to get crude alkaloids and the dry at 100°C.

Dissolve the alkaloidal residue in 10ml of 0.02N HCl and titrate the excess with 0.02N NaOH employing methyl red as an indicator.

Each ml of 0.02N HCl used is equivalent to 0.005784 gm of alkaloid calculated as hyoscyamine.

Result:———

The structure for hyoscyamine is:-

Vitali's Identification test

Place two drops of concentrated HNO_3 on a few mg of a solanaceous alkaloid(atropine, hyoscyamine, scopolamine, or stramonium), and on another evaporating dish a few mg of homatropine. Evaporate to dryness. Now moisten the various residues with a few drops of alcoholic KOH solution. Record the color change.

Results:————

A yellow color is obtained on treatment with nitric acid which changes to violet on treatment with alcoholic acid.

Explain the reason the homatropine reacted differently than the other samples in this group. *No violet color is produced as homatropine contain mandelic acid in place of tropic acid(present in hyoscyamine or atropine)*

Vitamins

Contents

Experiment 49

Vitamins

Vtamins are generally divided into two major groups: fat soluble and water soluble. The fat soluble ones, which are usually associated with the lipids of natural foods, include Vitamin A, D, E and K. The vitamins of the B complex and vitamin C comprise the water soluble group.

Vitamin A is an alcohol with high molecular weight know as retinol and is found only in the animal kingdom, occurring mainly as an ester with higher fatty acids in the liver, kidneys, lungs, and fat deposits. Viamin A in plants occurs as carotenes or carotenoid pi gments.

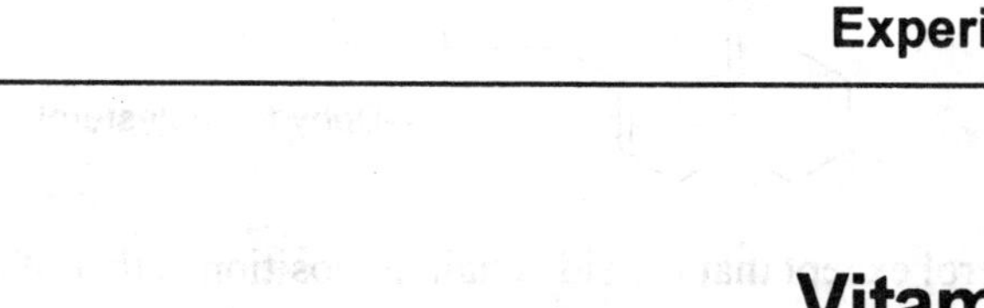

H3C
CH3
CH3
CH3
CH = CH-C = CHCH = CHC = CHCH2OH
CH3

Retinol

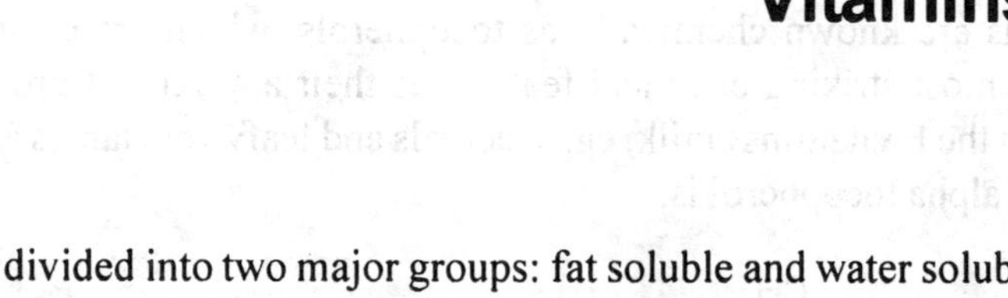

H3C
CH3
CH3
CH3
H3C
CH3
(CH = CH-C = CHCH = CHC = CHCH2)
CH3
H3C

β-Carotene

The D vitamins are actually a group of compounds known as sterols that occur in nature chiefly in animals. They include ergosterol (vitamin D2) and 7-dehydrocholesterol (vitamin D3). The structures for these are as follows:

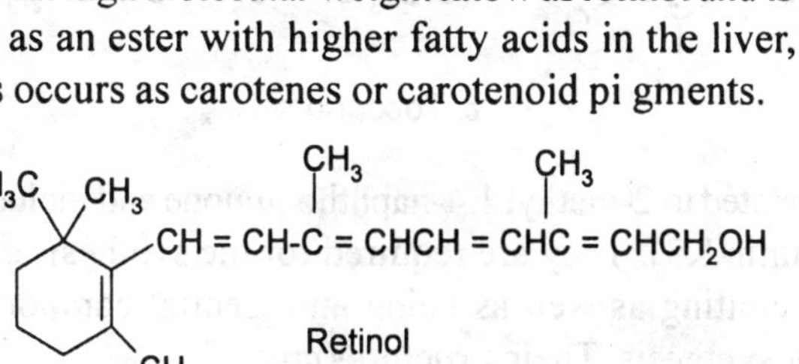

CH3
CH3
CH3
CH - CH2 CH =CH-CH-CH
CH3
CH3
H2C

Ergosterol

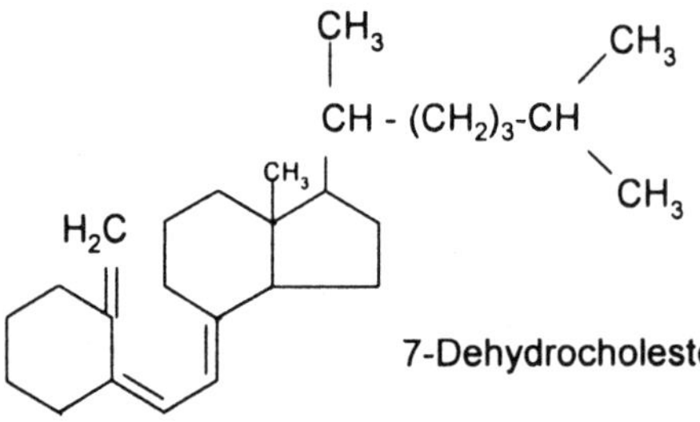

7-Dehydrocholesterol

It is same as ergosterol except that the side chain in position is that of cholesterol.

The E vitamins are known chemically as tocopherols, which are designated as α, β, and γ tocopherols. Their most striking chemical features is their antioxidant property. Wheat germ oil (particularly rich in the E vitamins),milk, eggs, cereals and leafy vegetables are sources for Vitamin E. The structure of alpha tocopherol is:

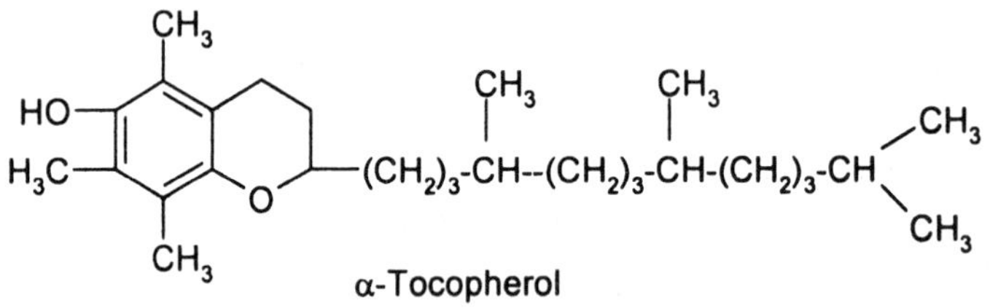

α-Tocopherol

The K vitamins are related to 2-methyl 1,4-naphthoquinone and include phytomenadione (vitamin K1) and menadione(vitamin K3). They are required for the synthesis of prothrombin in the blood, which promotes proper clotting as well as being an essential component of the phosphorylation process involved in photosynthesis. Their structures are:

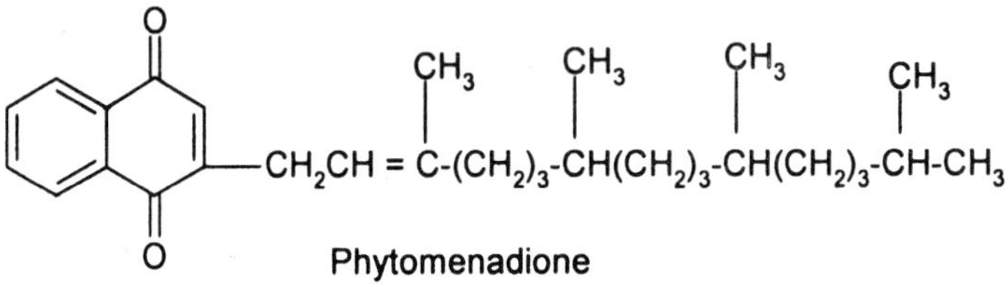

Phytomenadione

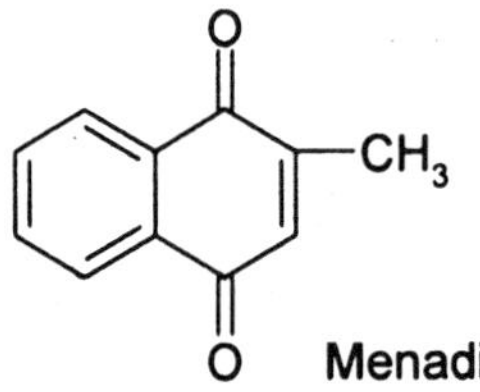

Menadione

The chemical structure of vitamin C (ascorbic acid) resembles that of a monosaccharide. Ascorbic acid functions as a reducing agent in both plant and animal tissues. Its structure is;-

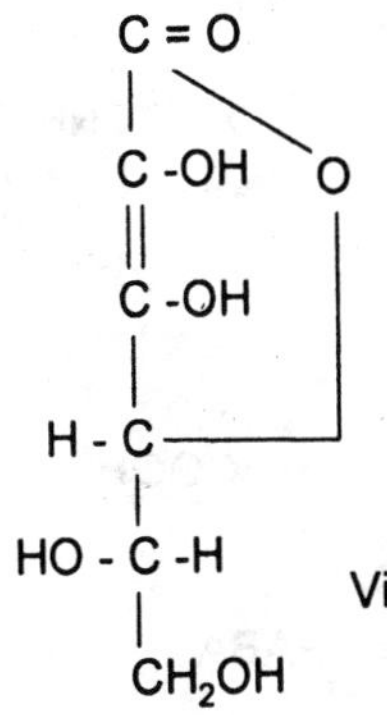

$$
\begin{array}{l}
C = O \\
| \\
C\text{-OH} \quad O \\
|| \\
C\text{-OH} \\
| \\
H\text{-}C \\
| \\
HO\text{-}C\text{-H} \qquad \text{Vitamin C (Ascorbic acid)} \\
| \\
CH_2OH
\end{array}
$$

The B vitamin complex includes the following:

Thiamine-B_1 Pantothenic acid

Riboflavin-B_2 Lipoic acid

Niacin Biotin

Pyridoxine-B_6 Para aminobenzoic acid

Folic acid-B_9

Cyanocobalamin-B_{12}

The structures of the vitamin complex are as follows:-

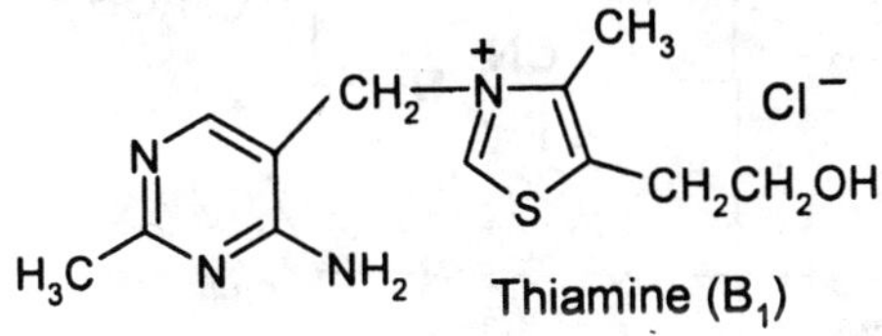

Thiamine (B_1)

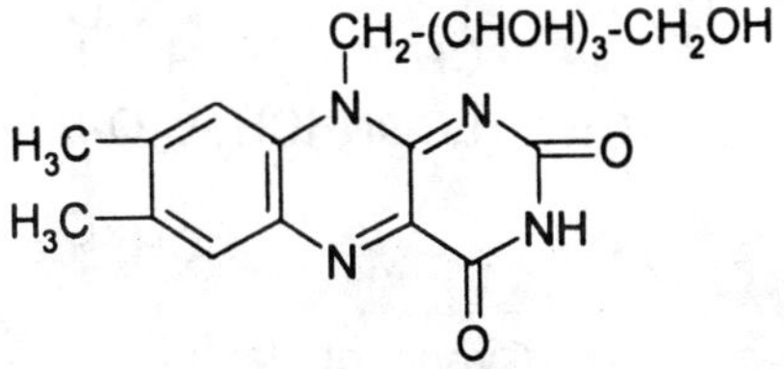

Riboflavin(B_2)

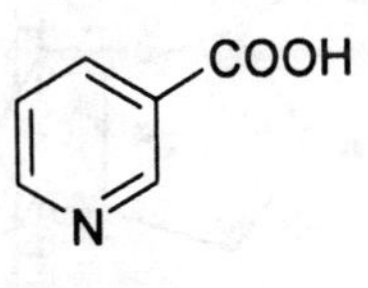

Niacin

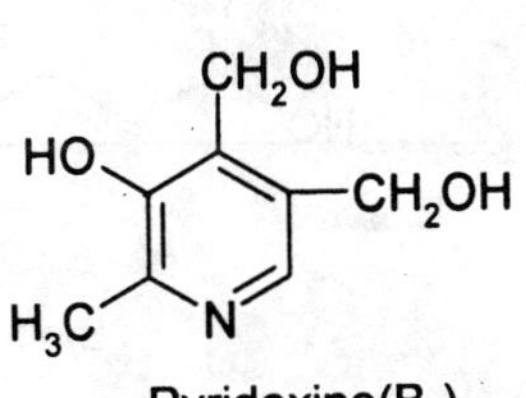

Pyridoxine(B_6)

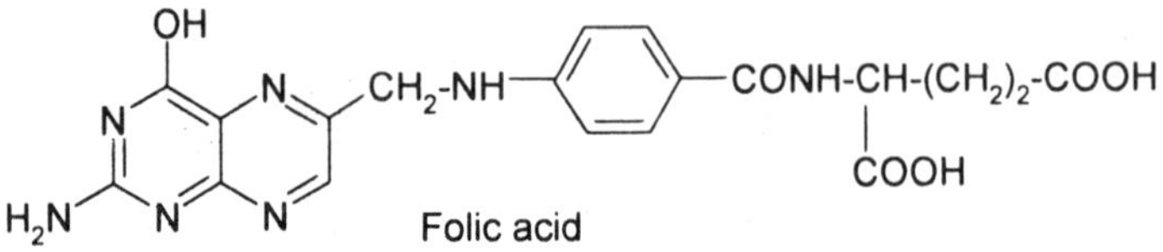

Folic acid

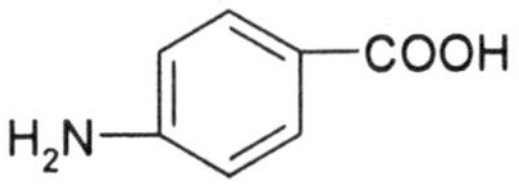

PABA

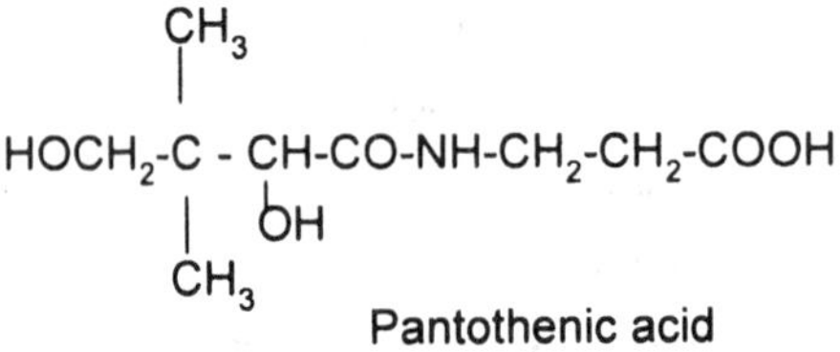

Pantothenic acid

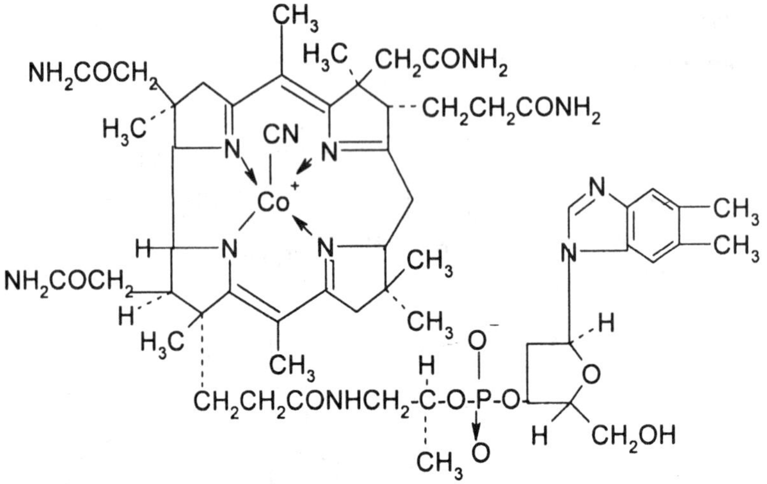

Cyanocobalamin

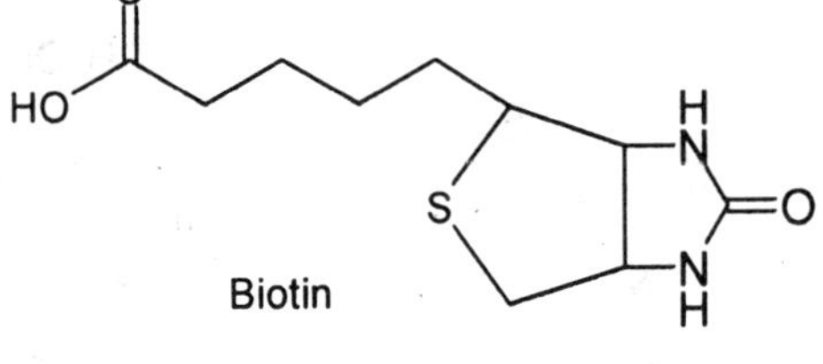

Biotin

Determining categories of vitamins is based on solubilities : In this experiment, you will make up a row of 12 test tubes, the first six of which will contain 10 ml of water and second six 10 ml of mineral oil. Number them 1 through 12. Into tubes 1 and 7 place 10 mg of riboflavin and shake each tube thoroughly. Record solubility results in the table. Repeat this procedure with the remaining vitamins listed and record results. Do your overall results confirm the traditional categories.

Vitamin	(Check)soluble	Insoluble
1. Riboflavin		
2. Ascorbic acid		
3. Ergosterol		
4. α-Tocopherol		
5. β-Carotene		
6. Thiamine		
7. Riboflavin		
8. Ascorbic acid		
9. Ergosterol		
10. α-Tocopherol		
11. β-carotene		
12. Thiamine		

Thiamine(B₁) as a Coenzyme

Thiamine is the first member of the vitamin B complex. It acts as a coenzyme, which means it must bond to an enzyme before the enzyme is activated. Without the coenzyme thiamine, no chemical reaction would occur. In this experiment, benzoin condensation of benzaldehyde is carried out using coenzyme, thiamine HCl as the catalyst.

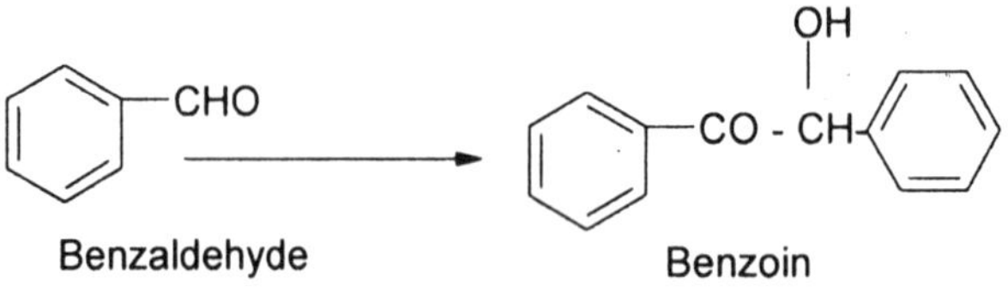

Benzaldehyde   Benzoin

Procedure

Add 1.5 gm of a thiamine HCl to a dry 50 ml flask and dissolve the solid in 5 ml of water by swirling. Add 15 ml of C_2H_5OH and cool the solution for a few minutes in an ice bath. Place a magnet in the flask, put it on a magnetic stirrer and add 5 ml of 2M NaOH. Now weigh the flask and solution. Then add 9 ml of benzaldehyde and reweigh to determine an accurate weight of benzaldehyde used. Attach an air condenser and heat the reaction mixture in a water bath at 60°C for 90 minutes.

At the end of the reaction time, allow the mixture to cool to room temperature and then induce crystallization of the benzoin by cooling the mixture in ice water. If the product separates as an oil, reheat the mixtre until it is once again homogeneous and allow it cool more slowly than before. When crystallization is complete, cool the mixture in an ice bath. Collect the product by vacuum filtration using a Buchner funnel and appropriate filter paper. Weigh the product and record all calculations.

Results :

Weigh of thiamine and benzaldehyde ——————— gm

Weigh of thiamine solution only(substract) ——— gm

Weigh of benzaldehyde ——————————— gm

Calculate the percentage yield :

Benzaldehyde   Benzoin

(106 m.w.)   (212 m.w.)

106/ gm = 212/ gm = ——— gm (theoretical yield)

% yield = Actual yield/theoretical yield × 100 = ———%

$$\frac{\text{Actual yield}}{\text{The oretical yield}} \times 100 = ...\%$$

Thiamine Assay of Vitamin B Complex Tablets

The object of this experiment is to determine the amount of thiamine as an ingredient of a multiple vitamin B complex tablet.

Thiamine (vitamin B) is non fluorescent compound but are estimated by fluorimetric method after oxidizing into fluorescent compound, thiochrome by alkaline potassium ferricyanide.

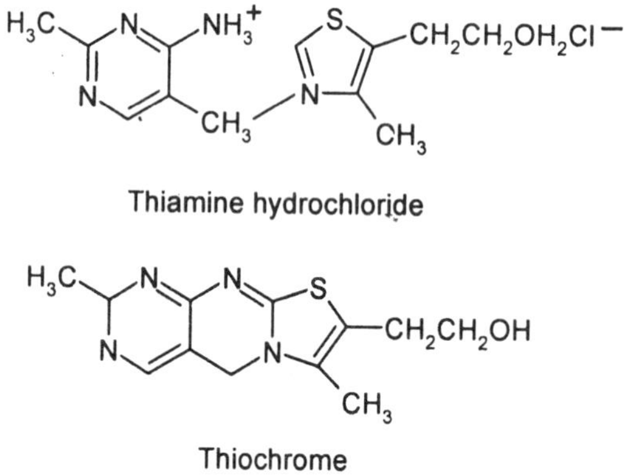

Thiamine hydrochloride

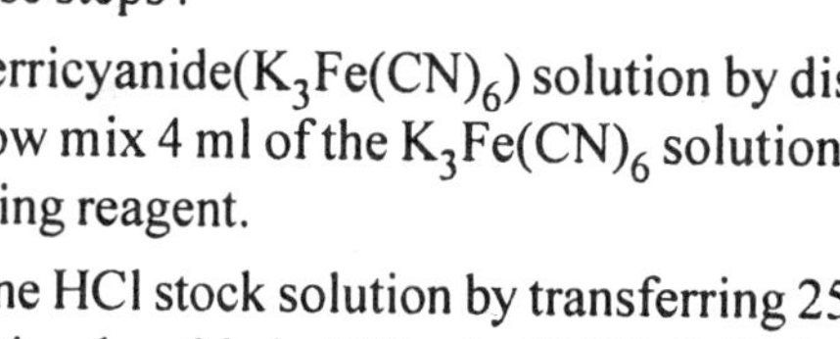

Thiochrome

It involves following precise steps :

1. Prepare a potassium ferricyanide($K_3Fe(CN)_6$) solution by dissolving 1 gm of the substance in 100 ml of water. Now mix 4 ml of the $K_3Fe(CN)_6$ solution with sufficient 3.5N NaOH to make 100 ml of oxidizing reagent.

2. Next, prepare a thiamine HCl stock solution by transferring 25 mg of thiamine HCl to a 1000 ml volumetric flask. Dissolve this in 300 ml of 20% C_2H_5OH whih has been adjusted with 3N HCl to a pH of 4.0. Now add the acidified alcohol to make up the volume.

3. To make the assay preparation, place in a suitable volumetric flask sufficient powder from the tablets to be assayed, such that when diluted to volume with 0.2N HCl, the resulting

128

solution will contain about 100 mg of thiamine HCl per ml. Now dilute 5 ml of this solution quantitatively and stepwise using 0.2 N HCl to an estimated concentration of 0.2 mg of thiamine HCl per ml.

4. The standard preparation is now made by diluting a portion of the stock solution, quantitatively and stepwise with, 0.2N HCl to obtain a preparation of 0.2 mg of thiamine HCl.

5. The next step is to take three test tubes of about 40 ml capacity and pipet 5 ml of the standard preparation while quickly (within 2 seconds) adding 3 ml of the oxidizing reagent and 20 ml of isobutyl alcohol, mixing by vigorous shaking. Now prepare a blank of the standard preparation in fourth test tube by substituting for the oxidizing agent an equal volume of the 3.5N NaOH and proceeding in the same manner.

Note: *Thiochrome has more solubility in Isobutyl alcohol.*

6. Repeat this procedure on the standard preparation with the assay preparation by taking 3 test tubes, including the making of a blank.

7. Next, into each of eight test tubes, add 2 ml of 100% C_2H_5OH and allow the phases to separate.

8. Decant to draw off 10 ml of the clear supernatant isobutyl alcohol solution into standardized cells. Then measure the fluorescence in a suitable fluorometer having an input filter of narrow transmittance range with a maximum of 365 nm and an output filter with a maximum of about 465 nm.

9. Calculate the m○g of thiamine HCl in each 5 ml of the assay preparation using the formula:

$$\frac{A-b}{S-d}$$

in which A and S are the average fluorometer reading of the portion of the assay and standard preparation treated with the oxidizing reagent and b and d are the readings of the blanks of the assay preparation and standard preparation respectively.

Note: Calibration curve may also be obtained by taking different concentration of standard solution and then concentration of unknown solution is read from this curve.

Determination of Vitamin C Content in Fruit Juices or in Commercial Tablets

A vitamin is an organic compound which must be obtained from the diet in order to maintaingood health. One such vitamin is vitamin C, ascorbic acid. All animal species except for primates (including humans), the guinea pig, the Indian fruit bat, and the red-vented bulbul bird, synthesize vitamin C for themselves. We, however, must obtain it from our food. Lack of vitamin C in the diet leads to a potentially fatal condition called *scurvy*. The recommendeddaily allowance of vitamin C for adults is 60 mg, but some scientists,especially the late Nobel prize-winning chemist Linus Pauling, believe that much more, up to several grams per day, should be taken. The structure of vitamin C is shown below.

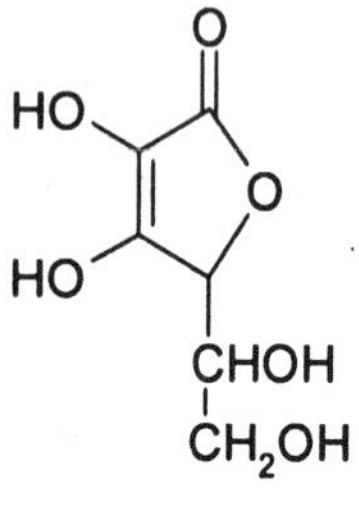

Vitamin C

Orange juice/lemon drink is probably the most widely consumed source today. Some people who wish to consume a large quantity rely upon vitamin C pills, for which the vitamin is usually produced bymicrobiological fermentation. "Organic" vitamin C can be isolated fromplant sources such as rose hips, at somewhat greater cost.

The vitamin has many roles in the body, not all of them well understood. One of its roles is as a water-soluble *antioxidant. Its reactivity as a reducing agent provides the chemical basis for our determination of vitamin C. The oxidizing agent which we will use to react with vitamin C is iodine. It is not practical to prepare standard solutions of iodine, however, because iodine is volatile and not very soluble in water. We will therefore generate the iodine in the presence of the vitamin C by the reaction:*

$$IO_3^- + 5\,I^- + 6H^+ \rightarrow 3I_2 + 3H_2O \tag{1}$$

As soon as molecular iodine forms, it will react with vitamin C according to:

Vitamin C
(Ascorbic acid) ·

Dehydroascorbic acid

$$\text{Vitamin C} + I_2 \longrightarrow \text{Dehydroascorbic acid} + 2H^+ + 2I^- \tag{2}$$

The product is sometimes called de-hydro ascorbic acid. (Note that the two hydroxyl groups on the five membered ring (C—OH) have been converted to carbonyl groups (C==O).When all of the vitamin C has been consumed, the excess iodine will react with iodide ion and starch indicator to produce a deep blue colored complex, which signals the end of the titration. This titration procedure is appropriate for testing the amount of vitamin C in vitamin C tablets, juices, and fresh, frozen, or packaged fruits and vegetables. The titration can be performed using just iodine solution and not iodate, but the iodate solution is more stable and gives a more accurate result.

There are **three** parts to this exercise. In the **first** part, you will titrate a pure vitamin C sample with potassium iodate (KIO_3) solution to determine the *titer value*. This is the *weight of vitamin C per volume of KIO_3 solution*. In the **second** part, you will analyze different juices or vitamin C pills and use the average titer value from the first part to calculate their vitamin C content. The **third** part will consist of your determining the vitamin C content of an unknown solid mixture, again using the average titer value from the first part.

Procedures

1. Drain a buret, rinse it with standard (about 0.01 M) potassium iodate (KIO_3) solution, and then fill it with the same solution. Be sure there are no bubbles in the tip of the buret. Record the exact concentration from the label.

2. Weighing by difference, *accurately* weigh about 0.1 gm (100 ± 20 mg) of pure vitamin C (ascorbic acid) into an Erlenmeyer flask. Add about 150 ml of distilled water to dissolve the solid.

3. Add the following reagents to the flask: about 5 ml of 1.0 M. HCl, about 10 ml of 0.60 M. potassium iodide (KI), and 10-15 (Starch solutions vary in their efficiency. Be sure to check onthe recommended value) drops of starch indicator. Take the initial buret reading and record it in your notebook.

4. Titrate the solution with the potassium iodate, adding small portions until the solution in the flask assumes a permanent blue color. Record the final buret reading. Calculate the titer value (mg vitamin C/ml KIO_3 solution).

5. Repeat steps 2-4 using another sample of vitamin C. If your titer values are consistent within 1%, you may proceed to step 6; otherwise, repeat until a consistent value is obtained. Since the analysis of your unknown depends on the accuracy of the titer value you determine, you may wish to repeat the determination of the titer of the KIO_3 solution a third time regardless of the agreement of the first two determinations.

6. **Unknown (Vitamin pill or fruit juice) :** This part of the exercise has you determine the percentage of vitamin C in a vitamin pill or fruit juice.

   (i) Weigh out or measure out the powdered tablet or juice respectively supposed to contain 100 mg of Vitamin C.

   For example, A certain juice indicates that one 8 fl oz serving contains the minimum daily requirement of vitamin C. How many ml of that juice will contain 100 mg of vitamin C?

   8 fl oz = 8 fl oz × 29.6 ml/fl oz = 240 ml

   This volume contains 60 mg. The volume of juice that contains 100 mg of vitamin C is 240 ml × 100 mg/60 mg = 400 ml

   We would need 400 ml samples of juice if we wished to titrate 100 mg of vitamin C in each titration.. Since we would wish to repeat the titration three times, we would need 3 × 400 ml, or 1,200 ml, or 1.2 l – i.e., more than one quart of this juice.

   (ii) Add the necessary reagents, and titrate as before. Since the unknowns vary widely in the percent of vitamin C, you may need to adjust the amount of unknown that you weigh out for subsequent determinations. Remember that the objective is to use about 25 ml of the potassium iodate solution to realize the full precision of the buret.

   Determine the amount of vitamin C in appropriate samples of the unknown by using the average value of the titer that you determined, and from that, the percentage of vitamin C in the unknown sample. Repeat this determination until you have at least two results that agree with each other to within 1%.

Observation

Titer Determination

	Run 1		Run 2		Run 3	
Mass of pure vitamin C		mg		mg		mg
Final buret reading		mL		mL		mL
Initial buret reading		mL		mL		mL
Net volume of titrant		mL		mL		mL
Titer value		mg/mL		mg/mL		mg/mL
Average titer value		mg				
Average Deviation mg/ml						

Identification of Unknown

	Run 1	Run 2	Run 3
Initial mass of vial	_____ gm	_____ gm	_____ gm
Final mass of vial	_____ gm	_____ gm	_____ gm
Mass of unknown	_____ gm	_____ gm	_____ gm
Final buret reading	_____ gm	_____ gm	_____ gm
Initial buret reading	_____ gm	_____ gm	_____ gm
Net volume of titrant	_____ gm	_____ gm	_____ gm
Quantity of vitamin C in sample	_____ gm	_____ gm	_____ gm
Percentage of vitamin C in unknown	_____ gm	_____ gm	_____ gm
Average Percent
Average Deviation
Percent Deviation

Calculations

For example, 33.47 ml of a KIO_3 solution is required to titrate a 107.5 mg of vitamin C in a standard sample.

The titer of this KIO_3 solution is 107.5 mg/33.47 ml = 3.212 mg/ml

24.56 ml of this KIO_3 solution is required to titrate a 115.8 mg test sample of a vitamin C pill that weighs 647.0 mg

This sample of the pill contained 24.56 × 3.212 = 78.89 mg of vitamin C

The entire pill contained (647.0/115.8) × 78.89 = 440.8 mg of vitamin C

Similarly, calculation is made to calculate the content of Vitamin C in juice.

Estimation of Vitamin C in Tablet Using 2,6-Dichlorophenolindophenol

The oxidized form of 2:6-dichlorophenolindophenol is colored blue in alkali and red in acid, while the educed form is colorless. Ascorbic acid is oxidized by 2,6-dichlorophenolindophenol and at the end point ascorbic acid is completely oxidized, a drop of 2,6-dichlorophenolindophenol solution gives rose-pink color.

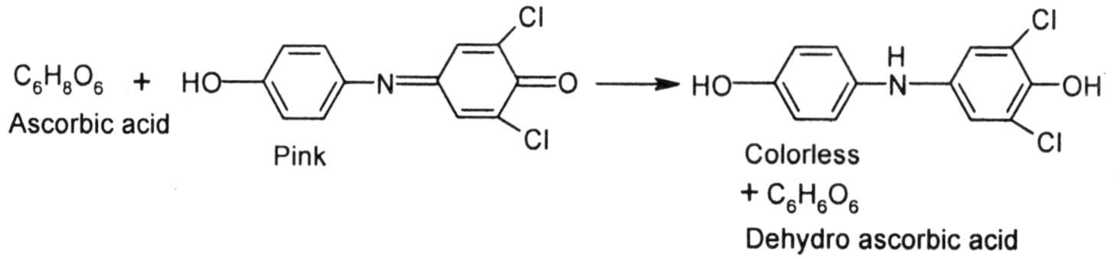

Procedure

(i) Measure accurately a volume equivalent to about 50 mg of ascorbic acid and transfer to a 250 ml volumetric flask.

(ii) Add 20 ml of solution of metaphosphoric –acetic acids, diute with water to 250 ml and mix.

(iii) Accurately measure a volume of dilution equivalent to about 2 mg of ascorbic acid into a 50 ml Erlenmeyer flask, add 5 ml of solution of metaphosphoric acetic acids and titrate with standard solution of 2:6-dichlorophenolindophenol, until the pink color persists for at least ten seconds, the titration occupying not more than two minutes.

(iv) Repeat the experiment with a mixture of 5.5 ml of solution of metaphosphoric acetic acids and 15 ml water, omitting the ascorbic acid. From the difference calculate the ascorbic acid in each ml of the injection.

Factor : Each ml of standard solution of 2:6-dichlorophenolindophenol= 0.1 mg of $C_6H_8O_6$

Metaphosphoric acid-Acetic Acids : Dissolve 5 gm of metaphosphoric acid in 40 ml of glacial acetic acid and add water to produce 500 ml. Store in a cool place and use within two days.

134

Colorimetric Method for Estimation of Riboflavin

Riboflavin is a water soluble vitamin. Naturally occurring riboflavin is yellow colored. Chemically, it is 7,8-dimethyl -10-(1-ribityl) isoalloxazine.

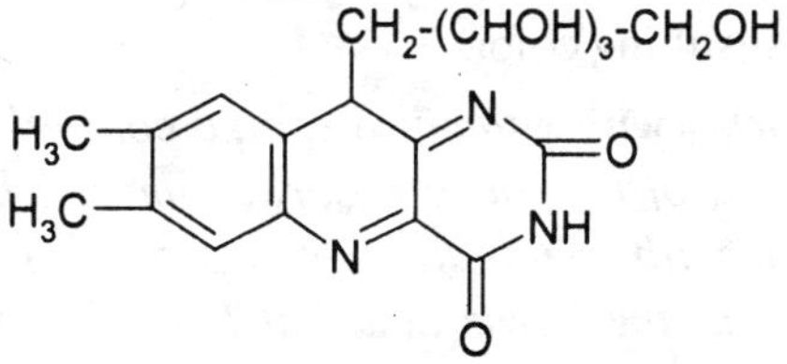

Riboflavin(B_2)

Method

1. Prepare a standard solution of riboflavin at a concentration of 190 mg/ ml in distilled water.
2. Transfer 1, 2, 3, 4, and 5 ml of standard solution to different test tubes.
3. Adjust the volume in each test tube to 10 ml with water.
4. Measure the absorbance values at 445 nm using a spectrophotometer against water as blank.
5. Plot a caliberation curve.
6. Then, weigh accurately a riboflavin(test sample) equivalent to 10 mg of riboflavin and mix with 70 ml of distilled water in a 100 ml volumetric flask.
7. Mix the contents to dissolve the sample and make up the volume to 100 ml anf filter.
8. Take 1 ml of the filtrate and analyse as done to make the calibration curve.
9. From the calibration curve, calculate the content of riboflavin.

Some Color Tests of Some Fat Soluble Vitamins

Retinol (Vitamin A): Prepare a 6 mg solution of retinol in chloroform by dissolving a 0.006 gm of retinol in 1 litre of the chloroform. Pipet out 1 ml of this solution into a small test tube and add 10 ml of $SbCl_3$ (if none in stock, you can make some by dissolving 20 gm of $SbCl_3$ in sufficient chloroform to make 100 ml). Observe the resulting color.

*Antimony tri chloride forms with vitamin A a blue colored complex **(Carr Price reaction)**. The first step is the conversion of retinol to a carbenium ion by $SbCl_3$. The carbenium ion is converted to anhydrovitamin with elimination of a proton. The addition produces a charge separation over the molecule of the Lewis acid $SbCl_3$ to the terminal C-C double bond (C_{15}) leads to the formation of a complex with the absorption maximum $\lambda_{max} = 619$ nm. On the other hand a complex with the absorption maximum $\lambda_{max} = 586$ nm is produced by addition of $SbCl_3$ to the endocyclic C-C double bond (C_4). The strong inductive effect of the chlorine atoms.*

The antimony trichloride reacts with the carotenoid to form a blue complex that can be measured by colorimetry.

Vitamin D_2 and D_3 tablets come as a mixture of ergocalciferol and cholecalciferol, which give identical color reaction. Place 0.5 mg of the tablet in 5 ml of chloroform, then add 0.3 ml of acetic anhydride and 0.1 ml of concentrated H_2SO_4. Observe the resulting color change.

Note : The initial color is not the final one on this.

Both compounds in chloroform are identified by the change in the color of the reaction mixture. The description of the change in color is as follows: a red color develops and immediately changes to green through purple and blue. Chloroform is used in the test only as a solvent to dissolve ergocalciferol and cholecalciferol in all the standards described above, so it should be possible to replace it with another solvent. Diethyl ether, ethyl acetate, n-hexane, toluene, and xylene were assessed as possible replacements for chloroform. The color of ergocalciferol and cholecalciferol in the reaction mixture with diethyl ether and ethyl acetate solutions was between lemon yellow and pale bluish-green. The reaction mixtures with n-hexane, toluene, and xylene as solvents formed emulsions when shaken, and the sulphuric

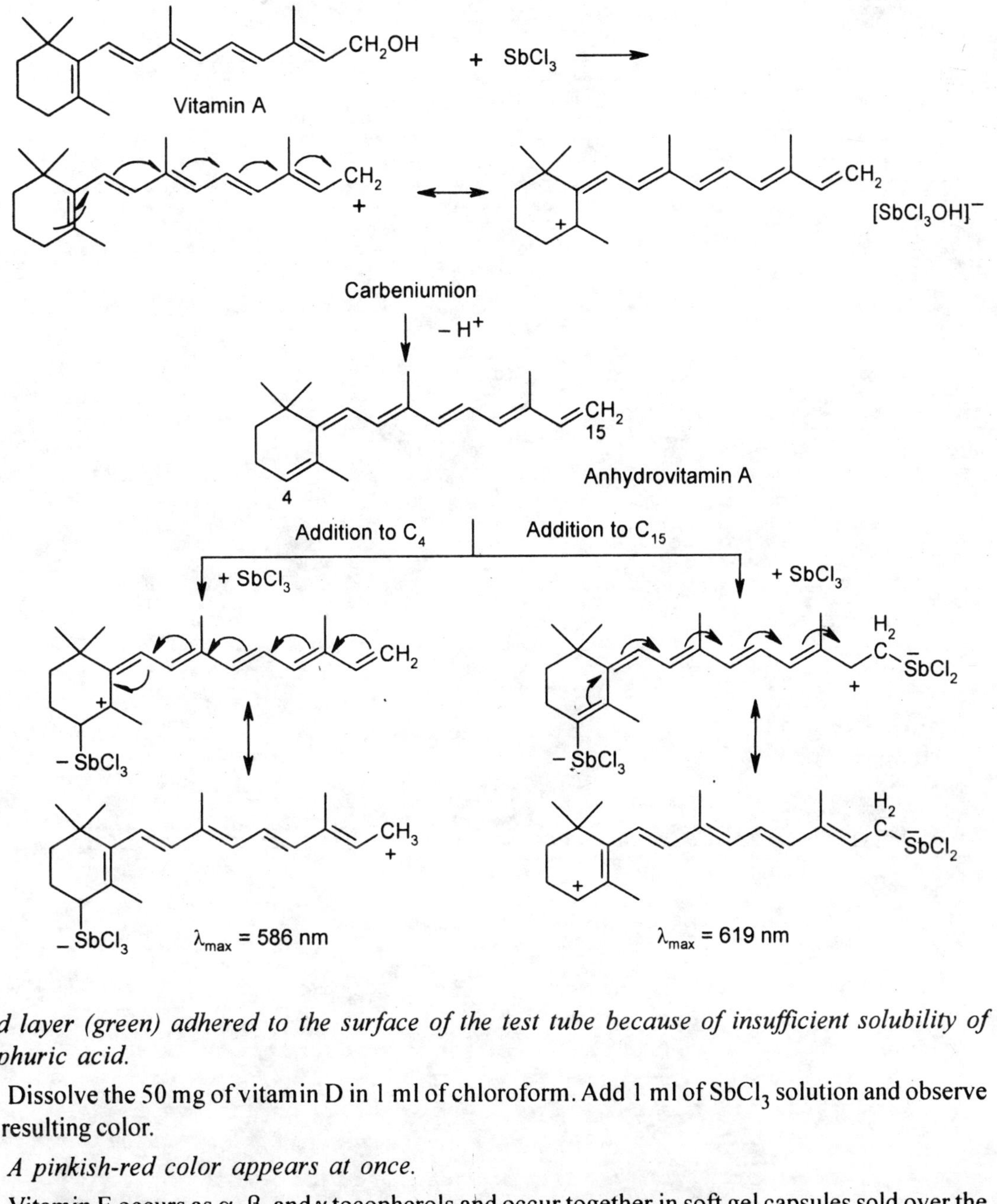
CH2OH
+ SbCl3
Vitamin A
CH2
+
[SbCl3OH]−
CH2
+
Carbeniumion
− H+
CH2
15
Anhydrovitamin A
4
Addition to C4
Addition to C15
+ SbCl3
+ SbCl3
CH2
− SbCl3
H2
C
SbCl2
+
− SbCl3
CH3
+
− SbCl3
λmax = 586 nm
H2
C
SbCl2
+
λmax = 619 nm

acid layer (green) adhered to the surface of the test tube because of insufficient solubility of sulphuric acid.

Dissolve the 50 mg of vitamin D in 1 ml of chloroform. Add 1 ml of $SbCl_3$ solution and observe the resulting color.

A pinkish-red color appears at once.

Vitamin E occurs as α, β, and γ tocopherols and occur together in soft gel capsules sold over the counter in pharmacies. The characteristic color reaction of tocopherol can be achieved by taking 10 ml of the vitamin E and adding 2 ml of concentrated HNO_3. Heat at 75^0C for 15 minutes. Observe the rsulting color.

The color changes from yellow to brick red.

Steroids

Contents

Experiment **56**

Steroids

Steroids comprise a natural product widely distributed throughout the plant and animal world. Although, they have widely variant pharmacological actions, they are defined as compounds having cyclopentanoperhydrophenanthrene nucleus.

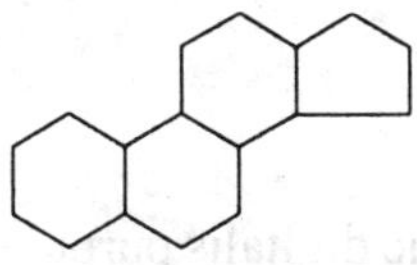

Steroids are included in such compounds as bile acids, cardiac glycoside, steroid hormones and vitamins. Some representative structures are shown here.

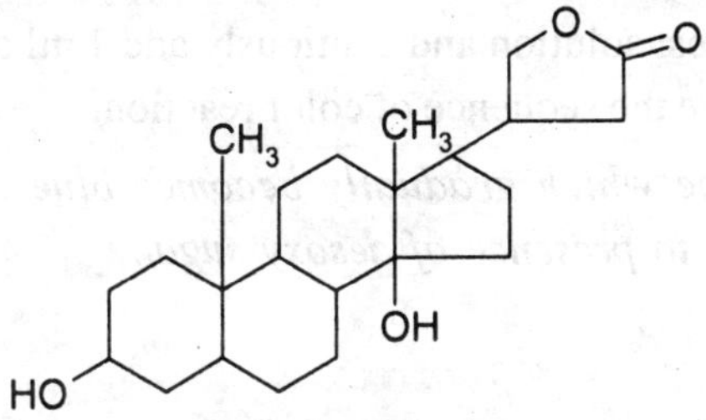

Digitoxigenin

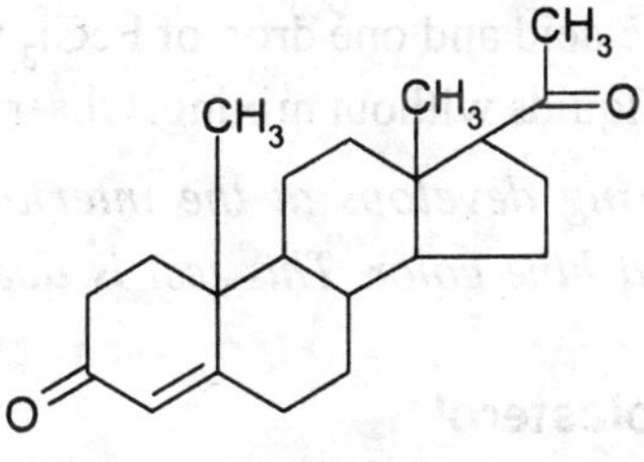

Progesterone

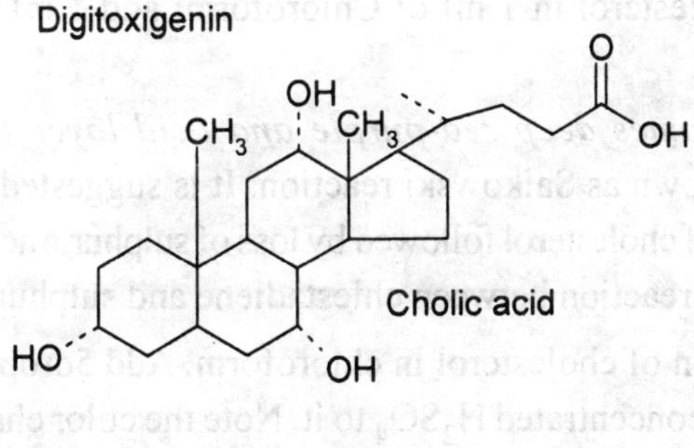

Cholic acid

Test for Hydrocortisone

Hydrocortisone is an example of a steroid that exhibits distinct color reactions to the treatment of reagents. It's structure is :

Hydrocortisone

Dissolve 2 mg of hydrocortisone powder in 2 ml of H_2SO_4 and allow it to stand for 15 minutes. Now dilute the solution with 10 ml of water and observe both color.

A green fluorescence is produced on adding sulphuric acid which becomes orange-red and finally dark red.

Test for Digitoxin

Digitoxin is a cardiac glycoside, obtained from the digitalis purpurea (purple foxglove) plant. Boil 1 gm of digitalis powder in 10 ml of 70% alcohol for 5minutes and filter. Dilute 5 ml of this with 10 ml of water and add 0.5 ml of lead acetate solution. To this, add 5 ml of chloroform and shake the mixture to separate out chloroform layer. Evaporate the chloroform layer to dryness. To this,add 2 ml of glacial acetic acid and one drop of $FeCl_3$ test solution and cautiously add 1 ml of sulphuric acid under the two liquids without mixing. Observe the sequence of color reaction.

A brown ring develops at the interface which gradually becomes blue and acetic acid layer aquires a blue color. This test is due to presence of desoxy sugar.

Test for Cholesterol

To a solution of 100 mg of cholesterol in 1 ml of Chloroform, add 1 ml of H_2SO_4. Observe the development of color.

*The chloroform layer becomes deep red-purple and acid layer takes on a deep green fluorescence.*This reaction is known as Salkowski reaction. It is suggested that mechanism of this reaction proceeds via sulphation of cholesterol followed by loss of sulphuric acid to yield cholestadiene. The red color is attributed to the reaction between chlestadiene and sulphuric acid.

Place 1 ml of a 0.1% solution of cholesterol in chloroform. Add 5drops of acetic anhydride to this. Mix well and add 1 drop of concentrated H_2SO_4 to it. Note the color changes and intensities for the first 5 minutes. *Blue or red color is produced.*

The final tests of this section are with the hormone estradiol whose structure is:

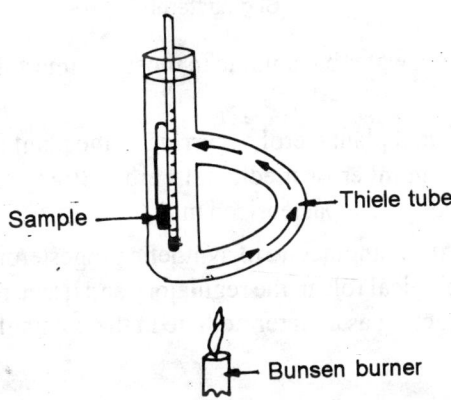

Estradiol benzoate

To about 2 mg of estradiol benzoate, add 3 drops of sulphomolybdic reagent (50 mg ammonium molybdate dissolved in 10 ml sulphuric acid). Add 1 ml of sulphuric acid and the 9 ml of water. Observe the change in color.

On adding sulphomolybdic reagent, a yellowish green color is obtained. This on adding sulphuric acid becomes pink with yellowish fluorescence.

Now dissolve 100 mg of estradiol benzoate in 10 ml of CH_3OH and add 100 mg of K_2CO_3 dissolved in 0.5 ml of water and reflux the mixture on a steam bath for 2hours. Add 30 ml of water and heat gently until all the alcohol is evaporated. Then, add 15 ml of water and keep the solution at a temperature of between 5 and 10°C for 1 hour. Filter the precipitate, wash it with cold water until the washings are neutral to litmus paper, and dry at 100°C for 1 hr.

Set up a meting point apparatus as shown in fig and determine the m.p. of the estradiol benzoate. *This sequence of treatment gives estradiol which melts at 175°C.*

Fig. 56.1. Determination of melting point.

57

Isolation of Stigmasterol from Soya Bean Oil

Stigmasterol is one of a group of plant sterols, or phytosterols, that includes beta-sitosterol, campesterol, ergosterol (provitamin D2), brassicasterol, delta-7-stigmasterol and delta-7-avenasterol, that are chemically similar to animal cholesterol.

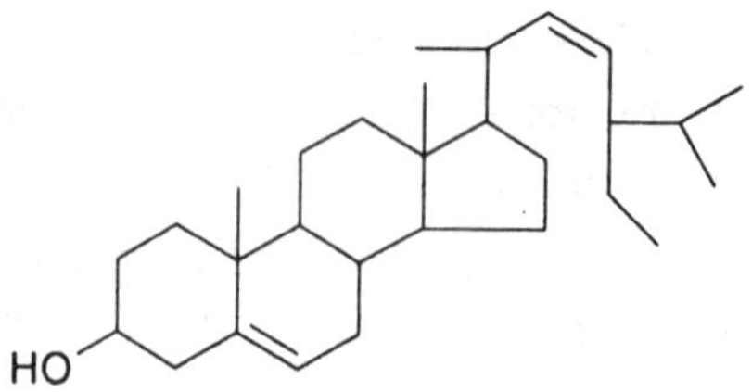

Stigmasterol

Phytosterols are insoluble in water but soluble in most organic solvents and contain one alcohol functional group.

Stigmasterol is an unsaturated plant sterol occurring in the plant fats or oils of soybean, calabar bean, and rape seed, and in a number of medicinal herbs. Stigmasterol is also found in various vegetables, legumes, nuts, seeds and unpasteurized milk.

It is used as a precursor in the manufacture of synthetic progesterone, a valuable human hormone that plays an important physiological role in the regulatory and tissue rebuilding mechanisms related to estrogen effects, as well as acting as an intermediate in the biosynthesis of androgens, estrogens, and corticoids.

Isolation procedure

1. Place 200 gm of Soya bean oil in flask and add to it 500 ml of absolute alcohol and 150 gm of KOH dissolved in minimum quantity of water.
2. Refux the contents for 2 hrs. Cool the flask, dilute with 500 ml of water and transfer the contents to a separating funnel.

3. Extract the contents twice with ether with 500 ml each.

4. Combine the ethereal extract and concentrate it one fourth volume.

5. Wash the ethereal extract with water until free from alkali.

6. Concentrate the alkali free extract and dissolve the residue in 250 ml of petroleum ether, pass steam until it is nearly saturated and then leave it overnight.

7. Collect the colorless crystal on a Buchner funnel, wash with cold water and dry. m.p. 140-142ºC.

Color reaction

To a few mg of compound in chloroform, add conc. sulphuric acid and acetic anhydride.Record the development of color.

A green colored solution is obtained.

Plant Acids

Contents

Plant Acids

Plant acids are defined as simple organic compounds containing not more than six carbon atoms and two or three carbonyl groups. Many of them function as intermediates in cellular respiration. Several, such as citric acid, malic acid and succinic acid, occur widely in plant tissues in rather high concentration. Others, less well known, that occur in smaller quantities include a-ketoglutaric aci and cis-aconitic acid.

Isolation of Citric acid from lemon

Citric acid is a weak organic acid found in citrus fruits. It is a good, natural preservative and is also used to add an acidic (sour) taste to foods and soft drinks. In biochemistry, it is important as an intermediate in the citric acid cycle and therefore occurs in the metabolism of almost all living things. It also serves as an environmentally benign cleaning agent and acts as an antioxidant.

Citric acid exists in a variety of fruits and vegetables, but it is most concentrated in lemons and *limes*, where it can comprise as much as 8% of the dry weight of the fruit.

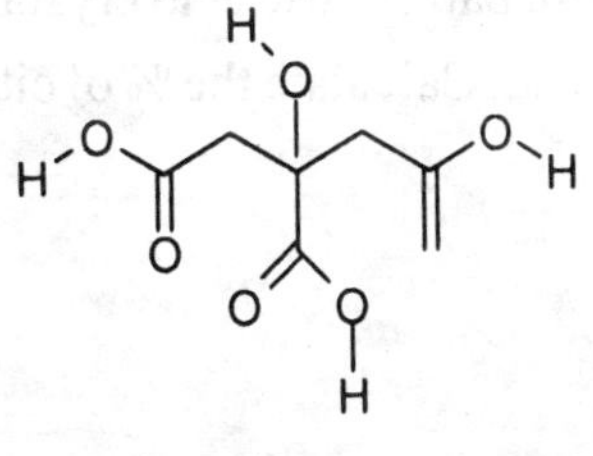

Citric acid's chemical formula is $C_6H_8O_7$ (structure shown at right). Its structure is reflected in its IUPAC name **2-hydroxypropane-1,2,3-tricarboxylic acid**.

The production technique, which is still the major industrial route to citric acid used today; cultures of *Aspergillus niger* are fed on sucrose to produce citric acid. After the mold is filtered out of the

149

resulting solution, citric acid is isolated by precipitating it with lime (calcium hydroxide) to yield calcium citrate salt, from which citric acid is regenerated by treatment with sulfuric acid.

It may be isolated from citrus fruits as the comparatively insoluble calcium salt. This compound displays unusual solubility properties in that it becomes less soluble at increased temperature. This information should be kept in mind when carrying out the following experiment.

(i) Measure 90 ml of frozen lemon juice concentrate into 250 ml beaker and carefully add a 10 % NaOH solution with stirring until solution is slightly alkaline. A distinct color change occurs at this point, the solution passing from a clear yellow to a brownish color.

(ii) Strain the solution through muslin to remove large particles of pulp and then filter through paper in a Buchner funnel. The pores of the filter paper may tend to become clogged by the extract inspite of previous straining. Should this occur, change the paper in the funnel once or twice as required to complete the filtration.

(iii) Measure the filtrate and record.

Result:—— ml

(iv) Now place the filtrate in a beaker and add 5 ml of 10% $CaCl_2$, stirring constantly for each 10 ml of filtrate. Heat to boiling and filter off the copious precipitate of calcium citrate($Ca_2C_{12}H_{10}O_{14}$) from the hot solution using a Buchner funnel.

(v) Wash the precipitate with a small quantity of boiling water. Now resuspend it in a minimum quantity of cold water, heat to boiling, and once more collect the insoluble $Ca_3C_{12}H_{10}O_{14}$ by filtration. Allow the salt to air dry. Wash and calculate the yield.

Calculation :

(vi) Citric acid may be prepared from the citrate salt by weighing the air dried salt and placing it in a beaker. Add sufficient 1N H_2SO_4 required to convert the salt to the acid. The equation for the reaction is:

$$Ca_3C_{12}H_{10}O_{14} + 3H_2SO_4 \longrightarrow C_{12}H_{10}O_{14} + 3CaSO_4$$

(vii) Allow the mixture to stand for a few minutes, filter off the insoluble $CaSO_4$, and evaporate to a small volume in a steam bath. Citric acid crystallizes out.

(viii) Filter, dry, and weigh the acid. Calculate the % of citric acid in the lemon juice sample used.

Determination of Molarity of
Acetic Acid in Vinegar

Vinegar occurs as the product of acetic fermentation of alcoholic products, usually wine, cider , or malt. The active principle principle of vinegar is acetic acid, which varies in amount from 2% to 15%. The formula for acetic acid is:

$$CH_3COOH$$

The amount of acetic acid in a sample of white vinegar will be determined in this experiment by titrating the vinegar with a solution of NaOH whose concentration is known. The indicator used is phenolphthalein.

Fill a burette with the 0.3N NaOH solution and pipet out 10 ml of the vinegar into a flask. Add 2 drops of the phenolphthalein indicator to the acid water mixture.

Record the molarity of the NaOH solution and the initial burette reading. Place the flask containing the vinegar under the burette and begin titration in increments of 1 ml while swirling in a magnetic stirrer. The titration is complete when the addition of about 1 ml of NaOH causes the color in the flask to change from colorless to a shade of pink. Record the burette reading at this point and substract the initial reading from this reading to ascertain the volume required for the approximate endpoint.

You should repeat this procedure two additional times to obtain an average or mean figure for the three titrations.

Results :

Sample number	1	2	3
Final reading	—	—	—
Initial reading	—	—	—
Volume of NaOH	—	—	—
Average of above three	—		

Molarity formula $M_1V_1 = M_2V_2$

(V_2= acid volume, which is 10 ml; M_2 = base molarity, which is 0.3; and V_2= average volume of base used)

Tannins

Contents

Tannins

Introduction

Tannins are one of the many types of secondary compounds found in plants

Characteristics of tannins

- oligomeric compounds with multiple structure units with **free phenolic groups**.
- molecular weight ranging from 500 to >20,000.
- soluble in water, with exception of some high molecular weight structures.
- ability to bind proteins and form insoluble or soluble tannin-protein complexes.

Tannins are usually subdivided into two groups :

- Hydrolyzable tannins (HT)
- Proanthocyanidins (PA) (often called Condensed Tannins)

Hydrolyzable tannins

HTs are molecules with a polyol (generally D-glucose) as a central core. The hydroxyl groups of these carbohydrates are partially or totally esterified with phenolic groups like gallic acid (→ **gallotannins**) or ellagic acid (→ **ellagitannins**). HT are usually present in low amounts in plants.

Some authors define two additional classes of hydrolyzable tannins: **taragallotannins**(gallic acid and quinic acid as the core) and **caffetannins** (caffeic acid and quinic acid).

Gallotannins

- The phenolic groups that esterify with the core are sometimes constituted by dimers or higher oligomers of **gallic acid** (each single monomer is called galloyl).
- Each HT molecule is usually composed of a core of **D-glucose** and 6 to 9 galloyl groups.

- In nature, there is abundance of mono and di-galloyl esters of glucose (MW about 900). They are not considered to be tannins. At least 3 hydroxyl groups of the glucose must be esterified to exhibit a sufficiently strong binding capacity to be classified as a tannin.

- The most famous source of gallotannins is **tannic acid** obtained from the twig galls of *Rhus semialata*. It has a penta galloyl-D-glucose core and five more units of galloyl linked to one of the galloyl of the core.

Ellagitannins

- The phenolic groups consist of **hexahydroxydiphenic acid**, which spontaneously dehydrates to the lactone form, **ellagic acid**.

- Molecular weight range: 2000-5000.

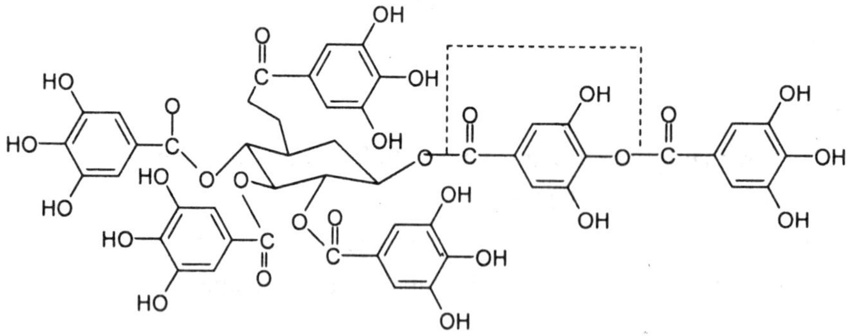

Gallotannin

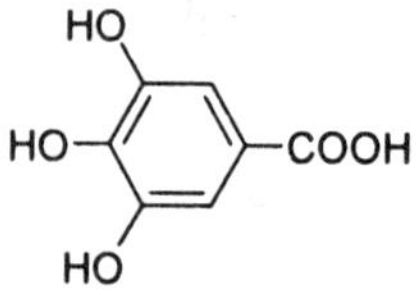

Gallic acid

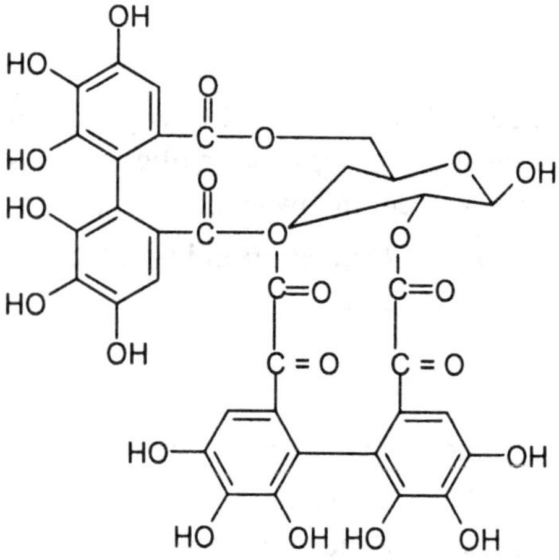

Ellagitannin

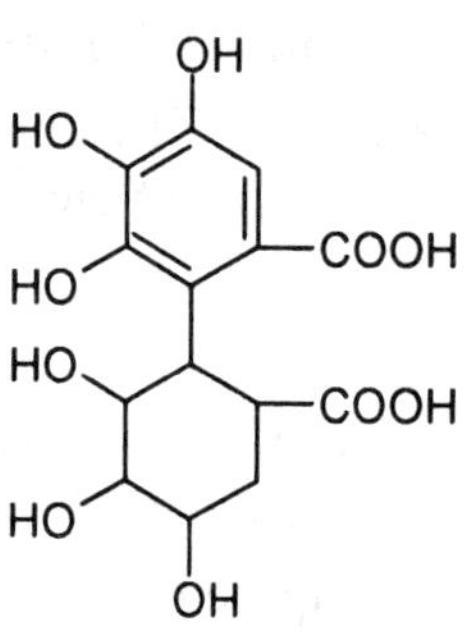

Hexahydroxydiphenic acid

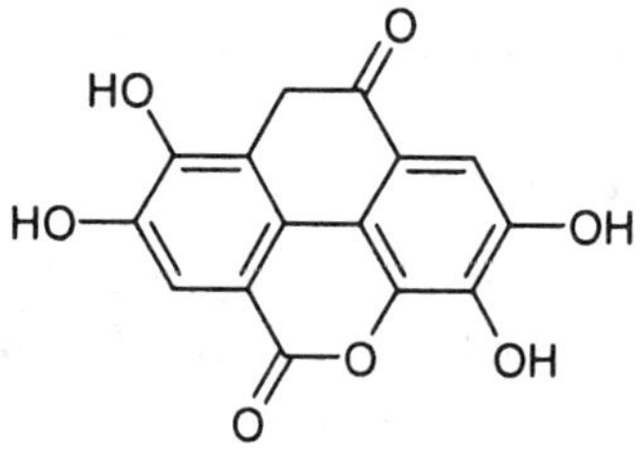

Ellagic acid

HT properties

- hydrolyzed by mild acids or mild bases to yield carbohydrate and phenolic acids
- Under the same conditions, proanthocyanidins (condensed tannins) do not hydrolyze.
- HTs are also hydrolyzed by hot water or enzymes (i.e. tannase).

Proanthocyanidins (condensed tannins)

PAs are more widely distributed than HTs. They are oligomers or polymers of flavonoid units (i.e. flavan-3-ol) linked by carbon-carbon bonds not susceptible to cleavage by hydrolysis.

- PAs are more often called **condensed tannins** due to their condensed chemical structure. However, HTs also undergo condensation reaction. The term, condensed tannins, is therefore potentially confusing.

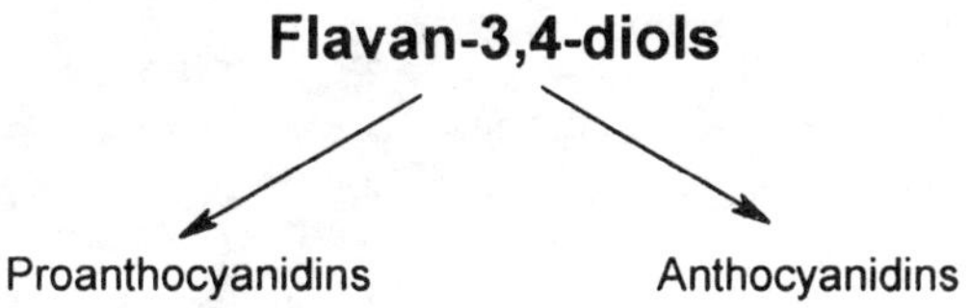

Flavan-3,4-diols

Proanthocyanidins   Anthocyanidins

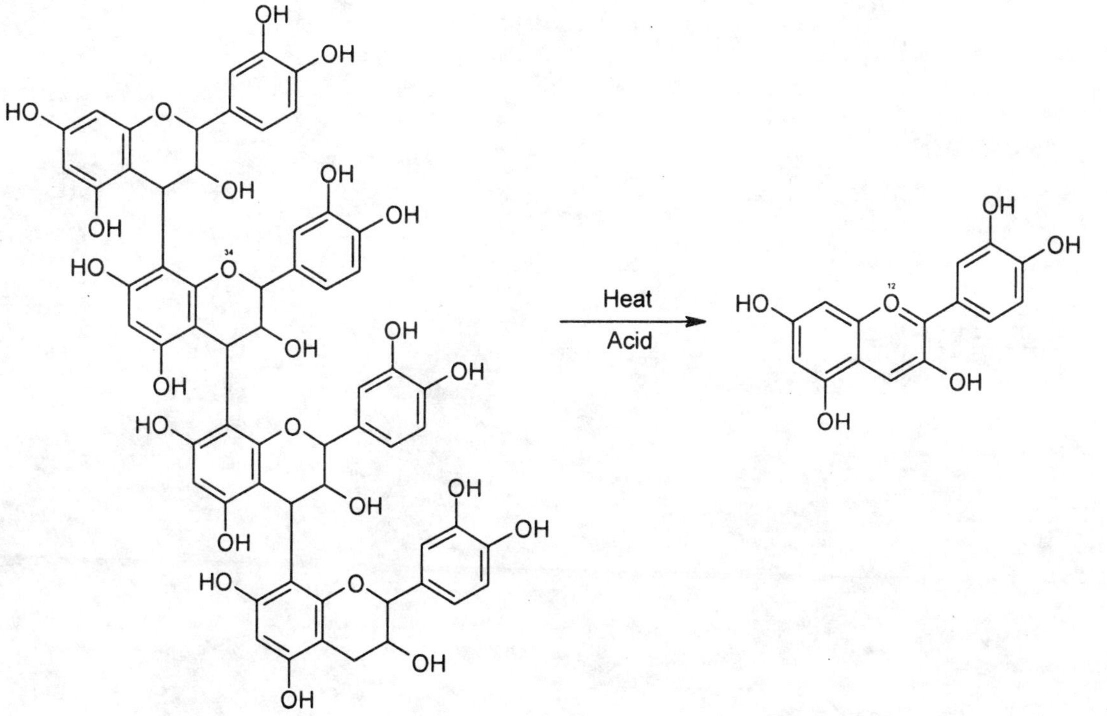

- The term, **proanthocyanidins**, is derived from the acid catalyzed oxidation reaction that produces red anthocyanidins upon heating PAs in acidic alcohol solutions.

- The most common anthocyanidins produced are cyanidin (flavan-3-ol, from procyanidin) and delphinidin (from prodelphinidin)

- PAs may contain from 2 to 50 or greater flavonoid units; PA polymers have complex structures because the flavonoid units can differ for some substituents and because of the variable sites for interflavan bonds.

- Anthocyanidin pigments are responsible for the wide array of pink, scarlet, red, mauve, violet, and blue colors in flowers, leaves, fruits, fruit juices, and wines. They are also responsible for the astringent taste of fruit and wines.

- PA carbon-carbon bonds are not cleaved by hydrolysis.

- Depending on their chemical structure and degree of polymerization, PAs may or may not be soluble in aqueous organic solvents.

61

Some Color Reactions of Tannins

Both classes of tannins are widely distributed in nature. Some examples are such substances as hamamelis leaf (with hazel) and nutgall, which have particular pharmaceutical significance as astringents and for the treatment of burns.

Other usable ways to distinguish tannins is to divide them categories of phlobotannins, which yield catechol and give reaction with ferric salts, and pyrogallotannins, which yield pyrogallol and give a blue color test with ferric salts.

Tannins are easily identifiable by color test. In this experiment, you will set up nine test tubes of about 40 ml capacity, labeled 1 through 9. The next step is to boil 1 gm of nutgall in 50 ml of water for 5 minutes. Cool and filter. Dilute 1 ml of the extract with 10 ml of water and place 1 ml of the nutgall extract in tubes 2 and 3. Next follow the same extraction, filtering, and diluting procedures for calumba root powder, which will be placed in tubes 4,5, and 6, and with oak bark, which will be placed in tubes 7,8, and 9. In tubes 1,4,and 7 place 10 drops of a 1% $FeCl_3$. In tubes 2,5,and 8 place 10 drops of a 1% solution of $Pb(C_2H_5O_2)_2$ and in tubes 3,6, and 9 place 10 drops of a 1% solution of quinine.

Record all observation in the table below, making particular note of color reactions and precipitates that occur. Make an estimate of the class of tannins that predominates in each of the extracts, keeping in mind the facts that most naturally occurring are mixture of both classes.

	Extract	Reagent	Observation	Class
1.	Nutgall	$FeCl_3$	–	–
2.	Nutgall	$Pb(C_2H_3O_2)_2$	–	–
3.	Nutgall	Quinine	–	–
4.	Calumba	$FeCl_3$	–	–
5.	Calumba	$Pb(C_2H_3O_2)_2$	–	–

(Contd.)

	Extract	Reagent	Observation	Class
6.	Calumba	Quinine	–	–
7.	Oak bark	$FeCl_3$	–	–
8.	Oak bark	$Pb(C_2H_3O_2)_2$	–	–
9.	Oak bark	Quinine	–	–

Some plants with tannins content of particular importance include :

Botanical name	Common name	Tannin
Castanea dentate	Chestnut	Tannic acid
Hamamelis virgiana	Witch hazel	Hamamelitannin
Krameria trianda	Rhatany	Catechol
Quercus infectoria	Nutgall	Tannic and gallic acid
Rosa gallica	Red rose	Pyrogallotannins
Uncaria gambir	Gambir	Catechutannic acid

The structure of catechin is:

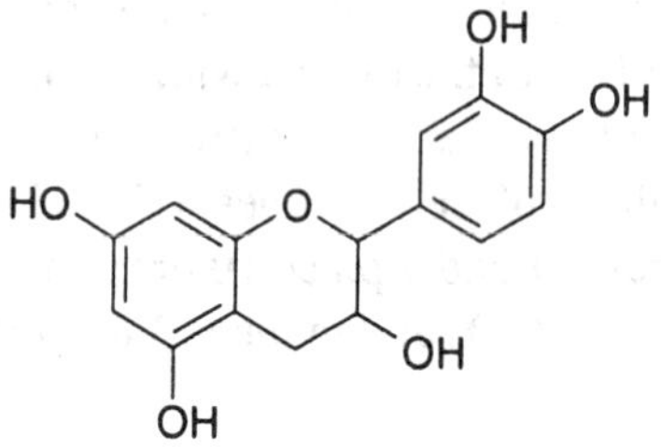

Isolation of Tannins from Terminalia Chebula (Myrobalan)

Terminalia chebula is a plant species belonging to the genous Terminalia, family Combretaceae. It is a flowering evergreen tree called in English the black myrobalan. It is also known as Haritaki (Sanskrit and Bengali), Harad (Hindi), Karkchettu (Telugu), Kadukkaya (Tamil), Harada (Marathi & Gujrati). It is native to Indian subcontinent and the adjacent areas such as Pakistan, Nepal and the South-West of China stretching as far south as Kerala or even Sri Lanka where it is called Aralu. The fruit of the tree has been used as traditional medicine for household remedy against various human ailments, since antiquity *Terminalia zeylanica van Heurck & Muell, Arg.* Terminalia chebula is rich in tannin. The chief constituents of tannin are chebulic acid, chebulagic acid, corilagin and gallic acid. Tannin of Terminalia chebula are of pyrogallol (hydrolyzable) type. A group of researchers found 14 components of hydrolyzable tannins (gallic acid, chebulic acid, punicalagin, chebulanin, corilagin, neochebulinic acid, ellagic acid, chebulegic acid, chebulinic acid, 1,2,3,4,6-penta-O-galloyl-H-D-glucose, 1,6,-di-O-galloyl-D-glucose,casuarinin, 3,4,6-tri-O-galloyl-D- glucose, terchebulin) from Terminalia chebula fruits.

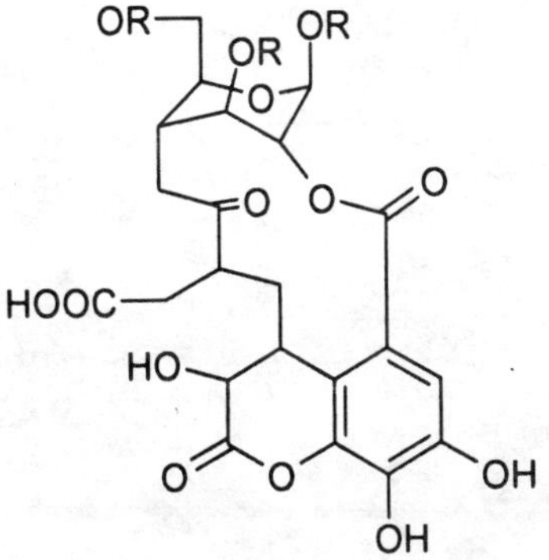

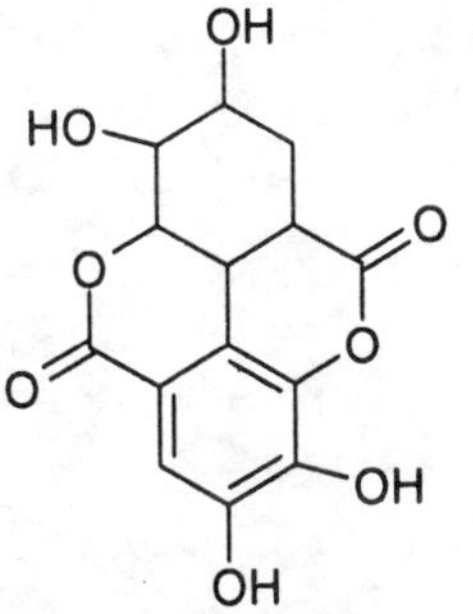

Galloyl Chebulinic acid (R= galloyl group)
Galloyl free Chebulinic acid(R =H)

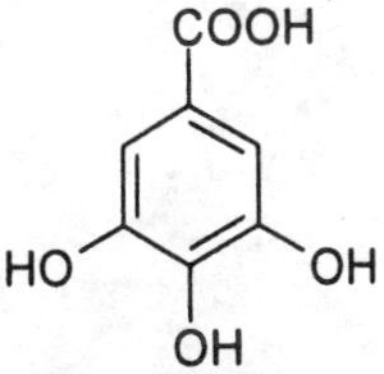

Ellagic acid

Gallic acid

Experimental Procedure

(i) Extract the powdered myrobalans (500 gm) with 95% ethanol (2 litres) on a shaker for 8 hrs.

(ii) Filter the extract and re–extract the marc with the ethanol (1 litre) for another 5 hrs. Filter, wash and combine the filtrate and washings.

(iii) Concentrate the extracts under vacuum. Dilute with distilled water and keep it overnight at 5°C.

(iv) Filter the extract and discard the flocculent precipitate.

(v) Extract the filtrate with equal volume of ethyl acetate three times.

(vi) Concentrate the combined ethyl acetate extract under vacuum to remove the solvent. Dry the tannins in a desiccator.

(vii) The yield is about 14%.

63

Determination of the Concentration of Polyphenolics in Apples

This can be accomplished by creating different concentrations of gallic acid (a specific type of polyphenolic) and then measuring their absorbance using a spectrometer. Then, use the standard to evaluate the polyphenolics filtered from an apple.

Introduction

Antioxidants are substances which have been shown to contribute to lowering the risk of developing chronic diseases and cancer. Such illnesses are caused by harmful free radicals within the body that attach to cells and cause them to mutate. Antioxidants are chemical substances which inhibit these harmful free radicals, thus preventing disease. Vitamin C is an example of one of these free radical inhibitors. By destroying free radicals and reducing cell damage, antioxidants can, as a group:

1. Boost the immune system

2. Prevent age related neurodegeneration

3. Prevent DNA damage (preventing cancer)

4. Prevent Cardiovascular disease (artherosclerosis, strokes, etc.)

Some foods with high concentrations of antioxidants are: beans, fruit, spinach, tomatoes, tea, wine, and chocolate. Consumption of food with antioxidants can help prevent the damage done by disease causing free radicals. Fruits, and more specifically apples, have been highly associated with the reduced risk of many chronic diseases and cancer, most likely due to their high antioxidant activity. In this lab experiment, we will be mainly considering the antioxidant content of apples. Within apples and other fruits, the majority of antioxidant activity derives from compounds, known as polyphenolics.

We will be extracting polyphenolics from a small sample of apples, and then observing the sample in a spectrometer to ultimately discover the concentration of polyphenolics within the apple. A spectrometer is an instrument used in the lab which measures the amount of light absorbed on a molecular level by different substances. The polyphenolics will react with Folin-Ciocalteau Reagent which acts as an indicator to absorb the light, and then the spectrometer will deliver an absorbance reading. The absorbance is proportional to concentration. The higher the absorbance, the higher the concentration will be. Once the absorbance of the sample of polyphenolics is determined, a graph of its standard will be used to relate it to concentration. This standard for polyphenolics must first be calibrated.

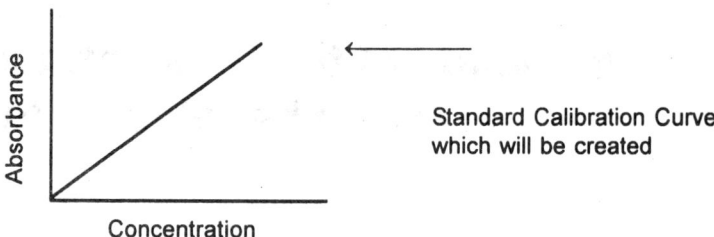

Materials

Part I : Polyphenolic extraction

- Knife
- Mortar and pestle
- Buchner funnel
- 125 ml funnel flask
- 50 ml volumetric flask

Part II : Polyphenolic standard

- 100 ml and 50 ml volumetric flasks
- 10 ml, 20 ml and 25 ml pipets
- 4-1 ml volumetric pipets
- 5 cuvettes
- Hot plate
- Spectrometer
- Thermometer and stand

Chemicals

Part I : Polyphenolic extraction

- Apple : approx. 10 gm
- 70% methanol : 75 ml

Part II : Polyphenolic standard

- Gallic acid : approx. 0.04 gm
- 70% methanol : 300-400 ml
- 7.5% sodium carbonate : 12 ml
- Folin-Ciocalteau reagent : 14 ml

Procedure

Preparation :

Part I: Polyphenolic Extraction

   A. Grind the Apple

      1. Cut approx. 10 gm of the apple into very fine pieces.

      2. Use a mortar and pestle to grind the apple with 10 ml 70% methanol for about ten minutes.

B. Filter

1. Vacuum filter the apple and 70% methanol mixture with a büchner funnel. Wash the mortar with minimum amount of 70% methanol. Use a beaker to press down on the apple mixture to release liquid contained in the apple flesh.

2. Once finished, pour filtrate into a beaker and wash the funnel with water and dry. Rinse the flask with 70% methanol.

3. Vacuum filter the retrieved mother liquor again through celite.

4. Retrieve the filtrate from the apple and dilute it to 50 ml using 70% methanol.

Part II: Polyphenolic Standard

A. Creating the Concentrations:

1. Create any four <u>different</u> concentrations of Gallic Acid using 70% methanol as the solvent. The concentrations should be between 0.015% and 0.001%.

$$\frac{0.015 \text{ gallic acid}}{100 \text{ ml } 70\% \text{ methanol}} \geq \text{concentration} \geq \frac{0.001 \text{ g gallic acid}}{100 \text{ ml } 70\% \text{ methanol}}$$

Do NOT make a dilution from a dilution.

1. Label and record all the solutions.

B. Set up the Heating Apparatus: The samples of the gallic acid concentrations will need to be heated.

1. Place a wire test tube rack within a glass basin and fill with water. Then place onto a heating plate with a thermometer submerged in the water.

2. Heat water to no higher than 60°C on a low setting (~3). Be patient and do not increase the temperature. While heating: Prepare the samples of gallic acid.

A. Prepare the solutions within 5 test tubes labeled Blank, 1, 2, 3, 4, and unknown (the apple).

1. The first sample will be a blank with no polyphenolics. In the test tube labeled "blank" add:

   a. 0.4 ml 70% methanol

   b. 1.6 ml 7.5% sodium carbonate (Na_2CO_3)

   c. 2 ml Folin-Ciocalteu reagent (add slowly)

2. In the test tube labeled "1" add:

   a. 0.4 ml concentration, 1

   b. 1.6 ml 7.5% sodium carbonate (Na_2CO_3)

   c. 2 ml Folin-Ciocalteu reagent (add slowly)

3. Repeat step 2b. in test tubes 2, 3, 4, and the unknown using concentrations 2, 3, 4, and the apple liquid.

B. Heat the samples:

1. Once the temperature of the water reaches 60°C, place the test tubes in the rack within the water and turn off the heat. If the water goes over 60°C before inserting the samples, use ice to bring the temperature down, then insert them. Heat the samples for exactly 5 minutes. While heating, fill the second basin with ice water.

2. After the 5 minutes, use tongs to remove the rack and place it in the ice water.

C. Reading the Absorbance

1. Transfer all the samples to cuvettes. *Do not label or mark the cuvettes.*

2. Place the blank sample in the Spectrophotometer. Be sure to wipe the cuvette clean of fingerprints and water drops.

3. Align the line on the cuvette with the line on the sample compartment of the Spectrophotometer.

4. Use the right knob to adjust the Absorbance to 0.

5. Insert samples 1-4 and record the Absorbance at 765nm.

Observation Data

Sample	Concentration	Absorbance
Blank	0%	0
1		
2		
3		
4		
Apple	Unknown	

Differentiation of Pale Catechu and Black Catechu

Pale Catechu (Gambier), a common ingredient used by Asians in chewing betel nut, is prepared from parts of the shrub *Uncaria gambier* (Uncaria gambir) of the family Rubiaceae. Traditional gambier is prepared by boiling the young leaves, pressing them to extract juice, making the juice into a concentrated form and drying it. There are different ways of moulding the final produce, in a block, cube or cake form. Different ways of boiling parts of the gambier plant result in different products of a varying taste. For example, the Chinese boil twigs over a prolonged period of time and make the end product as dry as possible resulting in a different kind of gambier. In India, rose water is mixed with cutch to make it aromatic and to give a more pleasant taste to the betel-quid. The traditional way to consume gambier is to apply it as a paste on betel leaves after mixing it with lime and water, wrapping the leaves with some betel nuts and chewing it. It has a mild narcotic effect and stains the mouth red. In Southeast Asia, gambier is sometimes chewed alone as a gum.

Black Catechu is an extract prepared from the wood of *Acacia Catechu* (family-Leguminosae). It is mostly used in tanning industry. Catechu is obtained by grinding the wood of the acacia catechu and boiling it in water for 12 hrs. The wood is removed from the water, and the extract is steamed until it forms the consistency of a syrup. At that time, the syrup is stirred and poured into molds. After drying, it is broken up into irregular pieces.

Differentiating Test

1. Extract the Pale catechu with acohol and add sodium hydroxide solution to it.
2. Add few drops of petroleum ether and shake and keep for some time.
3. Repeat the same with Blak Catechu.
4. Observe the fluorescence.

The pale catechu shows the green fluorescence due to presence of gambier which is absent in black catechu.

Resins

Contents

Resins

Resins are amorphous products with a complex chemical nature. They are usually found in schizogenous or schzolysigenous ducts or avities and are the end products of metabolism. They are complex mixtures of resin acids, resin alcohols, resinotannins, esters, and resenes.Numerous resins are used in medicine and pharmacy, including rosin, guaic, mastic, ginger, tolu balsam, Peruvian balsam, and benzoin. They are divided into four basic categories: oleoresins, oleo-gum-resins, balsams, and glycoresins.

Examples in each category include:-

Oleoresin- turpentine, copaiba, ginger, and capsicum

Oleo-gum-resin-asafoetida and myrrh

Balsams-benzoin, tolu, peru, and styrex

Glycoresin-jalap and podophylum

The first activity in this section will be to **prepare jalap resin from the crude jalap powder root**.

(i) Place 5 gm of the powder in a 250 ml Erlenmeyer flask and add 100 ml of a 50:50 mixture of methanol (CH_3OH) and water. Swirl to mix thoroughly.

(ii) Next set up a percolation apparatus as shown and percolate the jalap powder solution through the cotton into receiving beaker.

(iii) Place the beaker in a water bath and boil gently until you have concentrated the percolate to one fourth its original volume.

(iv) Next pour the concentrated percolate into hot water. This action results in a precipitate of jalap resin. Filter, dry and weigh.

(v) Calculate percentage of resin in the crude powder.
Calculation:

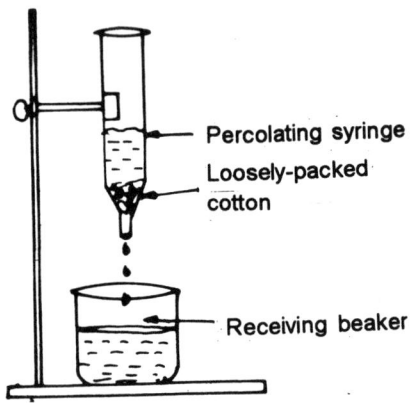

Percolating syringe
Loosely-packed cotton
Receiving beaker

Fig. 65.1. Percolation process.

Assay of Jalap

1. Place 10 gm of Jalap, in fine powder in 60 ml of mixture of 9 volumes alcohol and 1 volume of water in a flask. Digest the mixture on water bath under refluxing condition for 30 minutes. Transfer the warm mixture to a small percolator, allow it to drain, press the marc down gently, and percolate with warm alcohol mixture until 100 ml of the percolate, when cooled is obtained.

   (The Jalap is digested and percolated with alcohol to extract the resin completely)

2. Cool it and pipette out 20 ml of the percolate into a separator, add 40 ml of chloroform and 10 ml of HCl (about 1 in 100) and shake for 2 minutes. Alllow the mixture to separate, draw off the chloroform layer and extract the aqueous layer twice more, using 15 ml of mixture of 2 volumes of chloroform and 1 volumes of alcohol each time. Shake the combined Chloroform extract with 10 ml of HCl(1 in 100), again separate and wash the acid layer twice with 15 ml portion of chloroform and alcohol mixture.

   (The Jalap resin is insoluble in aqueous acid solution. It comes in the alcohol-chloroform mixture leaving non resinous constituents in the aqueous layer)

3. Pass the combined chloroform extract through the filter paper, moisted with chloroform-alcohol mixture.

4. Evaporate to dryness, add 2 ml of alcohol and again evaporate to dryness. Dry the residue to constant weight.

   The weight obtained represent the yield of total resin present in 2 gm of Jalap.

Some Color Reactions of Selected Resins

Some characteristic color reactions can be achieved with some of the resin.

Podophyllum resin : It consist of dried rhizome and roots of *Podophyllum hexandrum* Royale.

Add 0.5 gm of podophyllum powder in 5 ml of alcohol; then add 0.5 ml of 1N KOH and shake. Record the color.

Result:————————

A stiff jelly is produced

Myrrh : It is a red-brown resinous material, the dried sap of the tree *Commiphora myrrha*, native to Somalia and the eastern parts of Ethiopia.

Place 5 ml of tincture of myrrh in a small test tube and add 2 ml of concentrated HNO_3. Observe the color change.

Result:———

When triturated with water, myrrh yields a browish-yellow emulsion; with alcohol it yields a brownish-yellow tincture which acquires a purple tint on the addition of nitric acid.

Place 5 ml of tincture of myrrh in a small test tube and add 2 ml of bromine water. Observe the color change.

Result:——

A red coloration is produced.

Asafoetida : It is a oleo-gum resin, btained from the rhizome and roots of *Ferula foetida*.

1. Add nitric acid to asafetida resin and observe the resulting color.
    The drug gives green color.
2. Triturate about 0.5 gm of asafetida resin with sand and 5 ml of hydrochloric acid. To it, add little quantity of water, filter and to the filtrate add equal volume of ammonia solution. Observe the coloration.

A blue fluorescence is produced due to formation of umbelliferone from ferulic acid.

Gums

Contents

Some Chemical Features of Gums

Gums are natural hydrocolloids that may be classified as anionic polysaccharides or salts of polysaccharides. They may therefore be categorized under the heading of carbohydrates, but due to their special importance to biological and pharmaceutical chemistry, are being considered in their own special section.

Gums are amorphous and translucent substances that are frequently produced in higher plants as protectives after an injury. They are typically heterogeneous in composition and upon hydrolysis yield arabinose, galactose, glucose, mannose, xylose, and various uronic acids.

Gums find diverse applications in medicine and pharmacy, including dental adhesives, bulk laxatives, tablet binders, emulsifiers, gelating agents, stabilizers, and thickeners.

Gums, or hydrocolloids, can be summarized as follows:

1. Shrubs or tree exudates-acacia, karaya, tragacanth
2. Marine gums-agar, psyllium
3. Plant extracts-pectins
4. Starch and cellulose derivatives-ethyl and methyl cellulose
5. Microbial gums-dextran, xanthan

The varying stability of gums in dfferent solvents is an important consideration in pharmaceutical compounding. The first activity in this section will be designed to measure the relative solubilities of four gums in solutions of water, alcohol, and acid.

To begin the experiment, set up 12 flask each of 100 ml labeled 1 to 12 as shown in the illustration.

In flask 1,4,7 and 10, place 25 ml of water. In flasks 2,5,8,and 11, place 25 ml of 95% alcohol. In flasks 3,6,9,and 12, place 25 ml of 1N HCl.

The next step is to measure out 2 gm of acacia and add to flask 1. Repeat this procedure for flasks 2 and 3. In flasks 4,5, and 6, add 2 gm of gum tragacanth; in flasks 7,8, and 9, place 2 gm of gum karaya; and in flasks 10,11, and 12 2 gm of agar. When you have completed this, it will mean that each of the four gums will be tested with each of the three solvents.

You will need to shake each of the 12 flasks vigorously to achieve as much solubility as possible.

The next step is to set up a filtration funnel rack using previously weighed sections of cheesecloth and filter all the fluid mixtures. Record all original weights of the pieces of cheesecloth in the data section. Once filtration is complete, place the filters in a drying oven at 103^0C for 1hr. Remove from oven after the hour has passed, cool, and then weigh each filter and residue. Record data.

Calculate the weight of soluble material in each gum sample by substracting the original weight of the filter and residue.

Record data and calculation

Model for calculation:

Filter + residue weight = —— gm

Original filter weight = —— gm

Weight of insoluble material= —— gm

$$\% \text{ of insoluble gum material} = \frac{\text{wt. of insolubles}}{\text{Original wt. (2 gm)}} \times 100 = \% \text{ of insoluble material in each of the 12 solvent system}$$

100 – insoluble % = % of soluble material

Follow this pattern for calculation on all 12 systems.

Results:————

On the basis of your calculations, which of the following gums is:

The most water soluble? ————

The least water soluble? ————

The most alcohol soluble? ————

The least alcohol soluble? ————

The most acid soluble? ————

The least acid soluble? ————

(See identification test for gums for solubility behaviour).

Identification Tests for Gums

1. Acacia gum

Acacia is the dried gummy exudation from the stem and branches of Acacia senegal Willd. and of some other species of Acacia.

Identification

A. To 5 ml. of a 2 per cent w/v solution add 1 ml. of strong lead subacetate solution; a flocculent white precipitate is produced.

B. Dissolve 0.25 gm. in 5 ml. of water by shaking in the cold, add 0.5 ml. of hydrogen peroxide solution and 0.5 ml. of a 1 per cent w/v solution of benzidine in alcohol (90 per cent), shake and allow to stand; a deep blue color is produced.

C. Mount a small quantity, in powder, in ruthenium red solution, and examine microscopically; the particles do not acquire a red color (distinction from agar and from sterculia).

D. To 10 ml. of a 2 per cent w/v solution, add 02 ml. of a 20 per cent w/v solution of lead acetate; no precipitate is produced (distinction from agar and from tragacanth).

E. To 0.1 gm in powder add 1 ml. of N/50 iodine; the mixture does not acquire a crimson or olive-green color (distinction from agar and from tragacanth).

Solubility

It is nsoluble in alcohol (95 per cent).It is almost entirely soluble in an equal weight of water, yielding a translucent, viscous, slightly acid solution which is not glairy and, when diluted with more water and allowed to stand, does not yield a gummy deposit.

2. Gum tragacanth

Tragacanth is the dried gummy exudation obtained by incision from *Astragalus gummifer* Labill. and some other species of Astragalus.

179

Identification

A. To 4 ml. of a 0.5 per cent w/v solution, add 0.5 ml. of hydrochloric acid and heat for thirty minutes in a water-bath. Divide the liquid into two parts. To one part add 1.5 ml. of sodium hydroxide solution and 3 ml. of potassium cupri-tartrate solution, and warm in a water-bath; a red precipitate is produced. To the remainder of the liquid, add barium chloride solution; no precipitate is produced (distinction from agar).

B. To a 0.5 per cent w/v solution, add a 20 per cent w/v solution of lead acetate; a voluminous, flocculent precipitate is produced (distinction from acacia, from ghatti gum, and from sterculia).

C. Mount a small quantity, in powder, in ruthenium red solution, and examine microscopically; the particles do not acquire a pink colour (distinction from sterculia and from agar).

D. To 0.1 g., in powder, add 1 ml. of N/50 iodine; the mixture acquires an olive-green colour (distinction from acacia and from agar).

Solubility

It is sparingly soluble in water, but swells into an homogeneous, adhesive, gelatinous mass. It is insoluble in alcohol

3. Karaya gum

The dried gummy exudation from Sterculia urens and other species of Sterculia (Sterculiaceae)

Identification

A. Boil 1 gm of the sample with 20 ml of water until a mucilage is formed. Add 5 ml of hydrochloric acid and boil the mixture for 5 min. A permanent red or pink color develops.

B. Warm 0.5 gm of the sample with 2 ml of 5 M sodium hydroxide; a brown colour is produced.

C. Shake 1 gm of the sample with 80 ml of water for 24 h. Boil 4 ml of the resulting mucilage with 0.5 ml of concentrated hydrochloric acid, add 1 ml of 5 M sodium hydroxide and filter. To the filtrate add 3 ml of potassium cupric tartrate solution and heat. A red colored precipitate is formed.

Solubility

Gum Karaya, like Gum Tragacanth, does not dissolve in water to give a clear solution but rather forms a colloidal sol. Karaya gum swells in 60% ethanol distinguishing it from other gums. It yields a thick, syrup-like liquid. Gum Karaya will form viscous sols in hydroalcoholic solutions ranging up to 60% to 35% alcohol concentration.

4. Agar

It is dried gelatinous substance, obtained from Geldium amansi.

Identification

    A. Boil 1.5 gm with 100 ml water until solution is effected and then cool at room temperature. A stiff jelly is produced.

    B. To a 0.2 per cent w/v solution, add 1 ml of hot solution of tannic acid, no ppt is produced(distinction from gelatin).

Solubility

Practically insoluble in cold water but soluble in boiling water. It is Insoluble in alcohol.

The Mucilage-Swelling Factor in Gums

The mucilage-swelling factor is an important physical characteristic of gums useful in medicinal preparations.

1. To test this feature, take three 50 ml beakers (graduated) and place 2 gm of plantago(psyllium) seed in the first, 2 gm of carrageenin(Irish moss) in the second, and 2 gm of gum in the third beaker.

2. Now measure out 40 ml of water in a small graduated cylinder and add it to the first beaker. Repeat this procedure for remaining two beakers.

3. Next place a stirring mangnet in each beaker and place each over a mangnetic stirrer and run for 12 hrs.

4. At the end of this period note the mucilage level of each beaker and record results.

   1. Plantago——————— ml
   2. Carrageenin————— ml
   3. Guar gum————————— ml

Check some references in pharmaceutical chemistry and explain how the mucilage-swelling may be a consideration for the compounding of various medicinals.

Determination of Total Ash and Acid Insoluble Ash Value of Gums

Ash value

Take about 2 or 3 gm, accurately weighed acacia gum in a tarred silica dish previously ignited and weighed. Scatter the ground drug in a fine even layer on the bottom of the dish. Incinerate by gradually increasing the heat- not exceeding dull red heat-until free from carbon. Cool and weigh. Repeat this procedure till constant weight is achieved. Calculate the percentage of ash with reference to air dried drug.

Repeat this procedure with agar and karaya gum. Record the finding.

Gum acacia: % of ash

Karaya gum: —————

Tragacanth gum: ————

Acid insoluble ash

Boil the ash of acacia gum, as obtained above for five minutes with 25 ml of hydrochloric acid, collect the insoluble matter on ashless filter paper, wash with hot water, ignite and weigh. Calculate the percentage of acid insoluble ash with reference to air dried drug. Repeat the same procedure with other gums and record the findings.

Gum acacia: % of acid insoluble ash

Karaya gum: —————

Tragacanth gum: ————

Standard value

Gum	Total ash	Acid insoluble ash
Acacia	Not more than 4%	Not more than 1.0%
Agar	Not more than 6.5%	Not more than 0.5%
Karaya	Not more than 8.0%	Not more than 1.0%

Balsams

Contents

Balsams

Determination of Acid Value of Balsams

Balsams are resinous mixtures that contain large proportions of benzoic or cinnamic acid or both, or esters of these acids. The medicinal balsams include Peru balsam, tolu balsam, styrax and benzoin.

Peru balsam, also called balsam of Peru, is obtained from trees abundant along the coast of San Salvador in Central America. It was imported to Spain by early explorers via Lima, Peru, hence the name. It is a pathological product being formed to the tree that causes the balsam to exude from the exposed wood.

Tolu balsam is obtained from trees growing abundantly along the lower Magdalena River in Columbia but is also found in Venezuela and the west Indies. Like Peru balsam, it is also obtained by making incisions through the bark and sap wood.

Styrax or storex, is a balsam obtained from both oriental(Levant) and North American sources, the latter sometimes being called sweet gum. It has a very ancient history, being mentioned by Arab physicians in the twelth century. Most of the styrax used in pharmacy comes from Turkey.

A discussion of benzoin appears in the next experiment. In this experiment we wil perform-titrations to determine the acid values of Peru balsam, tolu balsam, styrax by following the same procedures with samples of each of three substances and recording the data.

Dissolve 1 gm of the substance being tested in 50 ml of methanol and add 0.5 ml of phenolphthalein. Titrate using biurette and mangnetic stirrer with 0. 1MN KOH and record the acid value.

Formula

$$\text{Acid value} = \frac{5.61 \times n}{W}$$

where   n = Volume of Potassium hydroxide solution consumed.

   w = Weight (gm) of substance or the oil taken.

	Acid value
Peru balsam	_____
Tolu balsam	_____
Storax	_____

The final step in this investigation is to check the acid value from the official book or text book of related subject.

72

Differentiation of Siam and Sumatra Benzoin

Benzoin is a balsamic resin obtained from two major sources which gives rise to its name, either Siam or Sumatra benzoin. Siam benzoin is obtained from trees growing in Thailand(formerly called Siam), and in Annam, whereas Sumatra benzoin comes from trees native to southeastern Asia and the East Indies. They first appeared in literature when mentioned by an Arab pharmacist in the fourteenth century it had become an object of Venetian commerce.

The use of Siam benzoin is confined almost entirely to the perfumery industry, whereas Sumatra benzoin finds much wider use in pharmacy.

The object of this experiment is to perform two tests that will provide ways of distinguishing the two products.

Dissolve 5 ml of Siam benzoin in 20 ml of ether and pour the solution into a porcelin dish. Add three drops of concentrated H_2SO_4 and record the results. Now repeat the procedure, this time using Sumatra benzoin and again record the results.

Siam benzoin color reaction ————————————

Sumatra benzoin color reaction ————————————

A deep brown color is produced in Sumatra benzoin. Siam benzoin gives deep purplish red color.

The second set of tests to distinguish between the two benzoins is to warm 500 mg of powdered Siam benzoin with 10 ml of $KMnO_4$ and gently warm. Record any noticeable odor. Repeat the procedure using Sumatra benzoin and record any evidence of odor.

Siam benzoin ————————————.

Sumatra benzoin ————————————

Odor of benzaldehyde is produced in case of Sumatra benzoin due to presence of more cinnamic acid.

In third test, add an alcoholic solution of ferric chloride to an alcoholic extract of the Siam and Sumatra benzoin in a separate test tube and observe the resulting coloration.

Siam benzoin gives a green coloration while Sumatra benzoin does not give this test.

The next step is to check the accuracy of your recorded results using some official books or texts related to subject.

Volatile Oils

Contents

Steam Distillation of Peppermint Oil

Steam Distillation of Peppermint Oil

Volatile oils are the odorous principles found in various parts. Because they evaporate when exposed to air at ordinary temperatures, they are called volatile or essential oils. They are generally immiscible with water, but are sufficiently soluble to impart their odor to water. They are usually soluble, however, in ether, alcohols, and other organic solvents.

Many volatile oils are used in medicinal preparations. These include peppermint, menthol, cardamom, rose, pine, orange peel, cedar wood, spearmint, clove, thyme, anise, eucalyptus, and others.

Steam distillation is a mean of separating and purifying organic compounds by volatilization. In this experiment, we will separate peppermint oil from its leaves using this method. Most compounds, regardless of their natural boiling point, will distill by steam distillation at a temperature below that of the pure boiling point. This has become a very effective means of separating volatile oils from natural sources, since it involves less heat and hence less risk of destroying the compound you seek to isolate.

Place 3 gm of peppermint leaves in a 500 ml flask containing 200 ml of water. Connect this to a steam generator as shown in the Fig. 73.1. The flask with the peppermint leaves and water should then be connected to a condenser and a receiving flask for the volatile oil. *Caution:* Make sure the safety pressure tube in the steam generator is below the surface of the water at all times to prevent excessive pressure and a possible explosion. Begin heating the water in the steam generator until the volatile condensate begins to appear in the receiving flask. Continue this process until no more condensate appears in the receiving flask. Discontinue heating, cool down, and measure the ml of peppermint oil collected.

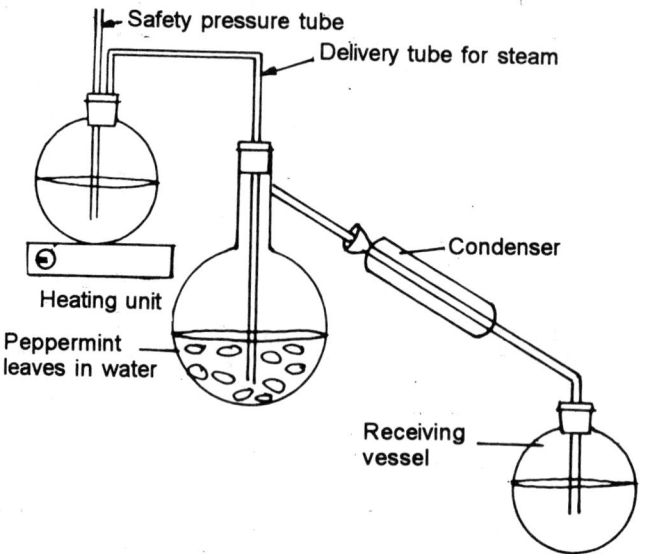

Fig. 73.1 Steam distillation assembly

Isolation and Characterization of Eugenol (Essence of Cloves)

Eugenol is isolated from cloves. The Clove tree is a tropical evergreen that develops clusters of flowers. These flower buds are collected and dried to give the familiar spice, used in cooking. The essential oil distilled from cloves (from *Eugenia caryophyllata*) is rich in **eugenol** (4-allyl-2-methoxyphenol; bp 250ºC), which is one of a class of compounds known as *phenols* (which are compounds containing a hydroxy-substituted benzene ring). **Caryophyllene** is also present in relatively small amounts, along with other terpenes. Eugenol is responsible for giving cloves their distinctive aroma and taste. The structure of eugenol is shown below.

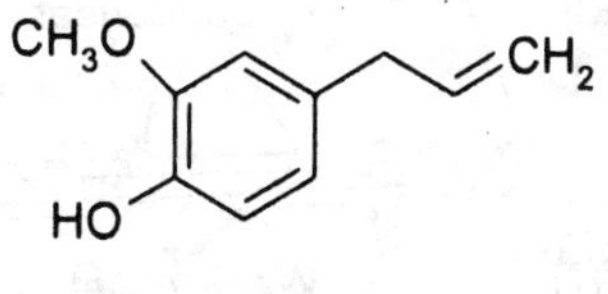

Eugenol

Experimental procedure

(i) Grind up whole cloves with a mortar and pestle to a powder. Weigh out 5.0 gm of this powder and placeit in a 500 ml round-bottom flask along with 150 ml of water, and a magnetic stir bar.

(ii) Assemble the apparatus for steam distillation as pictured below, and place a stir motor below the heating mantle. Whilestirring, heat the mixture using a Variac to control the rate of the distillation. A steady and even rate of distilling is better. During distillation, add small portions of water from the addition funnel to the distillation flask to maintain the original volume in the distillation flask.

(iii) The distillate that collects in the receiving flask will contain two immiscible liquids, a large amount of water and a small amount of your organic product. This will often make it look cloudy (which is a goodsign).

(iv) Collect about 100 ml of distillate and then stop the distillation.

(v) Now disassemble the apparatus and empty the separatory funnel. Transfer the distillate into the empty separatory funnel.

(vi) Now extract the distillation mixture successively with two 25 ml portions of ether. Combine the upper the ether layers in a Erlenmeyer flask and dry the solution by adding anhydrous magnesium sulphate. Allow the solution to sit over the drying agent for roughly 10 minutes.

(vii) Filter the liquid into a beaker. Carefully evaporate the ether on a steam bath in the fume hood, using a wooden stick to prevent bumping. When only 1-2 ml of solution remains, transfer the liquid into large pre-weighed vial with a pipet. Now resume heating on a steam bath until only an oily residue remains in the vial, which is eugenol.

(viii) Dry the outside of the vial and weigh it to determine how much eugenol was isolated from the cloves. Calculate the weight percentage of eugenol isolated form the cloves.

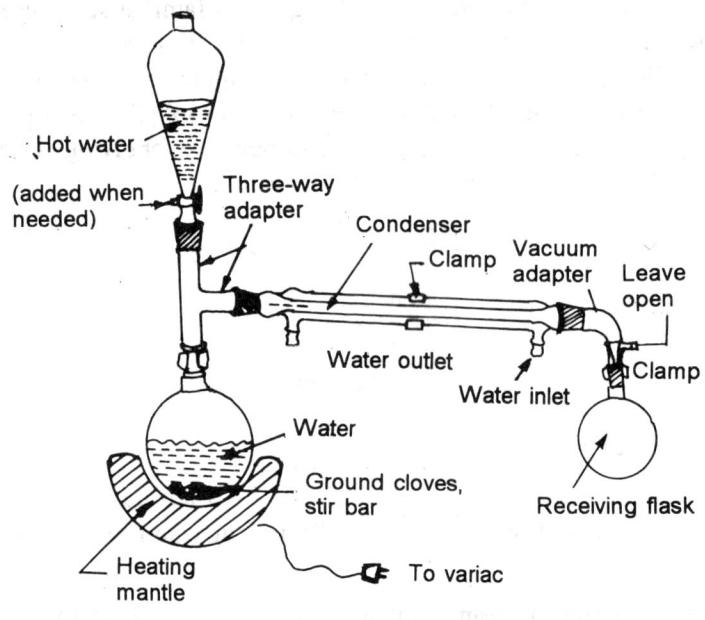

Fig. 74.1.

It was shown that about 7.5% of an oil could be recovered from cloves by steam distillation.

(ix) Perform the ferric chloride test or acquire an IR spectrum of your product. IR spectrum in functional group region shows the functional groups O-H (at 3560 cm^{-1}), sp^2 C–H (3080 – 3000 cm^{-1}), aliphatic C–H (2980 – 2940 cm^{-1}), and both alkene C = C (at 1640 cm^{-1}) and aromatic C = C (at 1514 cm^{-1}). Interpret the important stretches in the IR spectrum of eugenol in the non-fingerprint region.

Note : Why we didn't we purify eugenol by simple distillation, but instead used steam distillation.

The compound caryophyllene is another very abundant compound in cloves. It may be co-distilled during simple distillation and we obtained a mixture of this compound and eugenol.

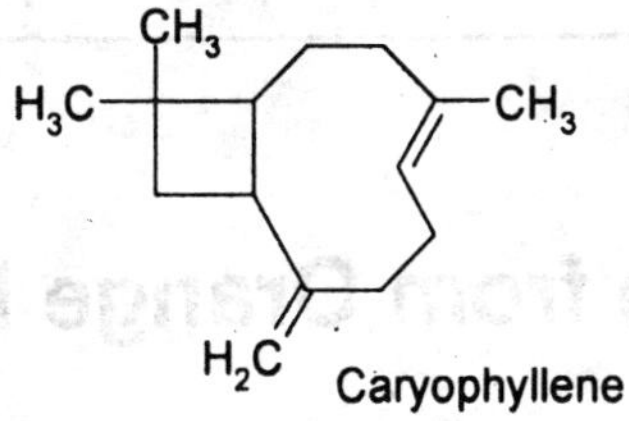

Caryophyllene

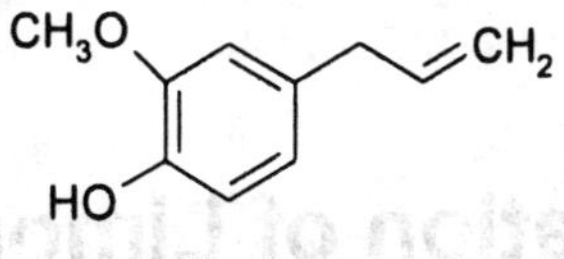

Eugenol

Isolation of Limonene from Orange Peels

(+) Limonene occurs in orange and lemon oils. The (-) form is present in the oil of peppermint whereas the racemic form, also known as dipentene, can be obtained from turpentine oil. (+) Limonene can be converted via its nitrosochloride into (-) carvone.

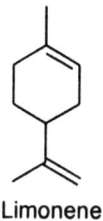

Limonene

Isolation procedure

1. Dry orange peels in the shade by spreading them out on a table.
2. Cut them into small bits and pack them in a Soxhlet extractor. Extract the material with light petrol (petroleum ether boiling at 40 – 60°C) till the siphoned material is colourless.
3. Remove the solvent by distillation on a water-bath and distil the residue under reduced pressure. Limonene distils over as a colourless liquid at 75°C at 27 mm pressure.

Alternatively, subject fresh orange peels to steam distillation and separate the essential oil distilling over. Dry the oil over anhydrous sodium sulphate and distil to obtain pure limonene. 100 gm of the crude essential oil yields on the average, 75 gm of pure limonene.

Estimation of Ciral in Lemon Oil

Lemon oil contain 4.5-5.0% Citral, the official requirement being not less than 4-0 per cent of aldehydes calculated as citral. Traces of other aldehydes, e.g. octyl aldehyde, monyl aldehyde, and esters, e.g. geranyl and linalyl acetates, are also present, and no doubt slightly modify the odour

Principle of Estimation

The estimation of citral (Aldehydes) is based on the fact that hydroxylamine combines quantitatively with aldehyde to form aldoximes :

$$C_9H_{15}CHO + H_2NOH.HCl \longrightarrow C_9H_{15}CHNOH + HCl + H_2O$$

Citral   Hydroxylamine   Citraldoxime
                  hydrochloride

    A known weight of oil is shaken in a stoppered tube with a known excess of an alcoholic solution of hydroxylamine hydrochloride which has been rendered first yellow* to methyl orange. The above reaction occurs partially with liberation of hydrochloric acid, and change in color to red. Semi-normal solution of potassium hydroxide is added to change the color to yellow. Upon further shaking, more aldehyde combines and the red color re-appears and is again discharged. This shaking and neutralization is repeated until the yellow color of the lower layer remains unchanged after 2 minutes of vigorous shaking, followed by separation of the oil, indicating that all the aldehyde has combined. The total volume of semi-normal solution of potassium hydroxide needed for the above processes is noted and gives an approximate value for the aldehyde. The test is repeated using as the standard for the end-point the reaction mixture obtained previously, to which a defined excess of semi-normal solution of potassium hydroxide has been added.

    The hydroxylamine HCl contains, as a result, a small proportion of free hydroxylamine. The latter is a weak base, the pH of the hydrochloride being 3-2. The orange color range of methyl orange lies between pH 2-9-4-0, hence if a neutral solution of hydroxylamine hydrochloride were used in the test, adjustment to the particular shade of orange corresponding to pH 3-2 would be necessary. This is difficult, hence a constant error is introduced by starting with a solution of hydroxylamine hydrochloride at about pH 9-0 (the pale yellow of methyl orange) and finishing at the same point—in this way an accurate end-point is obtained without affecting the result.

Hydroxyamine hydrochloride reagent : Dissolve 3.475 gm of $NH_2OH.HCl$ in 95 ml of 60% alcohol, add 0.5 ml of 0.2% methyl orange solution and sufficient alcoholic 0.5N KOH solution until yellow color is produced. Make up the volume to 100 ml with 60% alcohol.

Procedure

1. Weigh accurately about 10 gm of lemon oil in stoppered tube. Add to it, 7 ml of hydroxyamine HCl reagent in alcohol (60%) and a drop of methyl orange and shake well.

2. Titrate the liberated acid with alcoholic 0.5N KOH solution until the red color changes to permanent yellow in the lower layer.

3. Calculate the citral (aldehyde content) as follow :

   1 ml of 0.5N KOH solution = 0.07672 gm of citral

Preparation of 0.5 N alcoholic KOH solution : Dissolve about 35 gm of potassium hydroxide in 20 ml of water and add sufficient aldehyde free alcohol to make 1 litre. Allow the solution to stand in a tightly stoppred bottle(using either glass or a rubber stopper).

Estimation of Carvone in Caraway Oil

Carvone is a member of a family of chemicals called terpenoids. Carvone is found naturally in many essential oils, and is the principal constituent (50-70%) of the oil obtained from caraway seeds (*Carum carvi*).

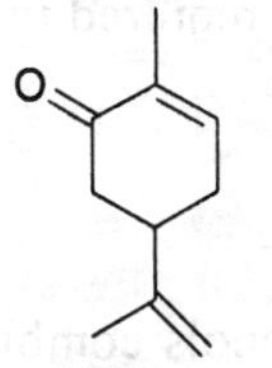

Carvone

Principle of Estimation

Ketones, like aldehydes, combine with hydroxylamine, and form ketox-imes. The method of estimating ketones follows therefore, in outline, that described for aldehydes.

Procedure

1. Weigh accurately about 1.5 gm of the caraway oil in a glass stoppered tube. Add to it, 10 ml of hydroxylamine HCl solution and place the tube in a water bath at 80^0C.
2. Titrate the solution with 1N KOH in 90% alcohol until the red color changes to yellow.
3. Continue the heating in water bath and at the 5minute interval neutralize the liberated acid with more alkali until the yellow color is obtained.
4. Calculate the Carvone content.

Factor : Each ml of 1N KOH solution = 0.1514 gm of carvone.

Note. This method gives an approximate value of carvone content. Hence, second determination should be carried out in exactly same manner using as the color standard for the end point determination. Calculate the carvone content of oil from the second determination.

Estimation of Eugenol in Clove Oil

Eugenol, is an allyl chain-substituted guaiacol, i.e. 2-methoxy-4-(2-propenyl) phenol. It is a clear to pale yellow oily liquid extracted from certain essential oils especially from clove oil, nutmeg, cinnamon, and bay leaf. It is slightly soluble in water and soluble in organic solvents. It has a pleasant, spicy, clove-like aroma. Clove oil is officially required to contain 85-0-90-0 per cent v/v of the phenol, eugenol.

Principle of Estimation

Estimation is based on the fact that phenols combine with caustic alkalis to form water-soluble compounds. Hence, the difference in volume between the oil used and that remaining uncombined represents the amount of phenol present in the portion tested. The estimation is carried out in a special flask, called a Hirschsohn or Cassia flask, which is stoppered and has a long neck graduated like a burette. The oil and alkali are shaken thoroughly for a prescribed period, and the uncombined oil is then raised to the graduated neck by the addition of more alkali. After standing for 24 hrs or more for complete separation to ensue, the volume of uncombined oil is read off. The percentage v/v of phenols is calculated from the data obtained.

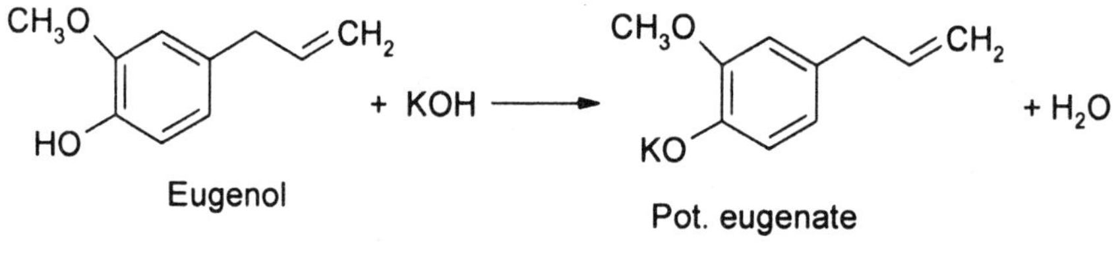

Eugenol + KOH ⟶ Pot. eugenate + H_2O

Procedure

1. Pipet 10 ml of clove oil into a 150 ml cassia flask, the neck of which is graduated from 0 to 6 ml at intervals of 0.01 ml.

2. Add 75 ml of KOH solution, shake the mixture for 5 minutes and heat for 10 minutes in boiling water bath, shaking the flask 3 times during the heating.

3. Remove the flask from a water bath and cool to room temperature.

4. When the liquids have separated completely, add sufficient KOH solution to raise the lower limit of the oily layer within the graduated portion of the neck.

5. Allow to stand for 24 hrs, the volume of the oily layer does not exceed 1.5 ml, indicating the presence in the oil not less than 85% by volume of total phenolic substances.

Note: If a 10 ml sample of oil yield 1.6 ml of residual liquid, then $10 - 1.6 = 8.4$ ml of eugenol dissolved and the percentage of eugenol in the sample:-

$$\frac{8.4}{10} \times 100 = 84\%$$

Assay of Peppermint Oil for Menthol content

Peppermint Oil is the volatile oil distilled with steam from the fresh overground parts of the flowering plant of *Mentha piperita* Linn (Fam.Labiatae), rectified by distillation and neither partially nor wholly dementholized. It yields not less than 5.0% of esters, calculated as menthyl acetate ($C_{12}H_{22}O_2$), and not less than 50% of total menthol ($C_{10}H_{20}O$),free and as esters.

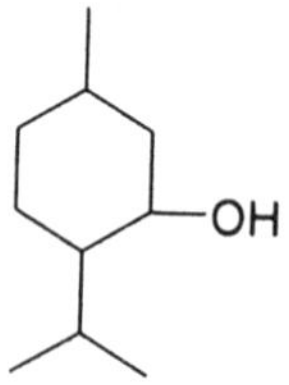

Menthol 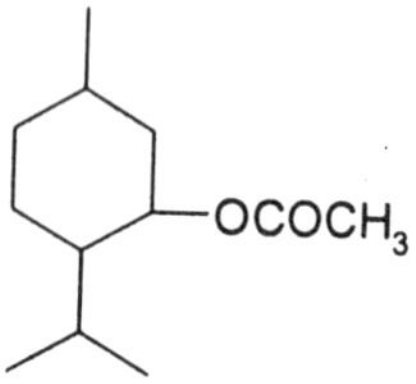   Menthyl acetate

Identification

Mix in a dry test tube 6 drops of Oil with 5 ml of a 1 in 300 solution of nitric acid in glacial acetic acid and place the tube in a beaker of boiling water: within 5 minutes the liquid develops a blue color which, on continued heating, deepens and shows a copper-colored fluorescence, and then fades, leaving a golden-yellow solution.

Assay for total esters

1. Place about 10 gm of Oil, accurately weighed, in a 250 ml round bottom flask.
2. Add 10 ml of neutralized alcohol and 2drops of phenolphthalein TS, then add, dropwise, 0.1Nsodium hydroxide until a faint pink color appears.
3. Add 25.0 ml of 0.5N alcoholic potassium hydroxide, connect the flask to a reflux condenser, and heat on a boiling water bath for 1hr.

4. Allow the mixture to cool, add 20 mlof water, add phenolphthalein TS, and titrate the excess alkali with 0.5Nhydrochloric acid.

5. Perform a blank determination in a similat manner.

6. Calculate the % of menthyl acetate.

Each ml of 0.5N alcoholic potassium hydroxide consumed in the saponification is equivalent to 99.15 mg of total esters calculated as menthyl acetate ($C_{12}H_{22}O_2$).

Assay for total menthol

1. Place 10 ml of Oil in an acetylation flask of 100 ml capacity, and add 10 ml of acetic anhydride and 1 gm of anhydrous sodium acetate.

2. Boil the mixture gently for 1hr, accurately timed, cool, disconnect the flask from the condenser.

3. Transfer the mixture to a small separator, rinsing the acetylation flask with three 5 ml portions of warm water, and add the rinsings to the separator. When the liquids have completely separated, discard the water layer, and wash the remaining oil with successive portions of sodium carbonate, diluted with an equal volume of water, until the last washing is alkaline to phenolphthalein TS.

4. Dry the resulting oil with anhydrous sodium sulphate, and filter.

5. Transfer 5 ml of the dry acetylated oil to a tared, 100 ml conical flask, and weigh.

6. Add 50.0 mlof 0.5N alcoholic potassium hydroxide, connect the flask to a reflux condenser, and boil the mixture on a steam bath for 1hr, accurately timed.

7. Allow the mixture to cool, add 10drops of phenolphthalein TS, and titrate the excess alkali with 0.5N hydrochloric acid.

8. Perform a blank determination.

9. Calculate the percentage of total menthol in the Oil tested by the formula:

$$\% \text{ of methanol content} = \frac{7.813\,(1 - 0.0021\,E)}{B - 0.021\,A}$$

in which A is the result obtained by subtracting the number of ml of 0.5N hydrochloric acid required in the above titration from the number of ml of 0.5N hydrochloric acid required in the residual titration blank, E is the percentage of esters calculated as menthyl acetate ($C_{12}H_{22}O_2$), and B is the weight of acetylated oil taken (see step 6).

Glycosides

Contents

Glycosides

Glycosides are compounds that yield one or more sugars among the products of hydrolysis. The most frequently occurring sugar is β-D-glucose, although rhamnose, digitoxose, cymarose, and other sugars are also components of glycosides. When the sugar formed is glucose, the substance may be called a glucoside. However, because other sugars may be developed during the hydrolysis, the term glycoside is used.

Chemically, the glycosides are acetals in which the hydroxyl of the sugar is condensed with a hydroxyl group of the nonsugar component and secondary hydroxyl is condensed within the sugar molecule itself to form an oxide ring. An example is the glycoside prunassin:

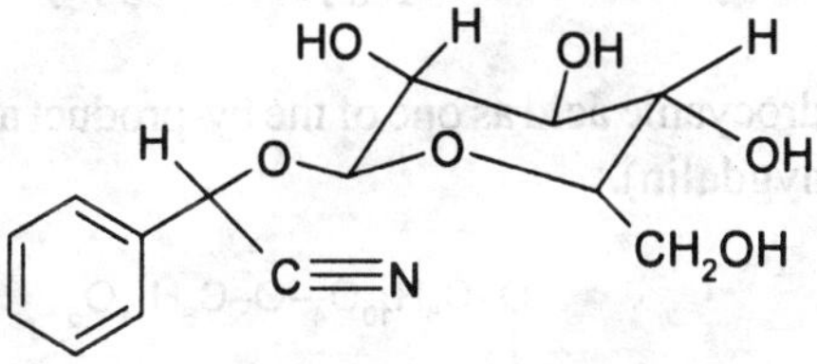

While glycosides are extremely difficult to categorize due to their complex and variant structure, the most workable current scheme seems to be the following:

1. Cardioactive glycosides-so called because of their action on the cardiovascular system. They include Digitalis(digoxin, digitoxin), Strophanthus(strophanthidin), and Squill(scillaren A and scillaren B).

2. Anthraquine-usually employed as cathartics and include Cascara(cascaroside A, B &C), Aloe(barbaloin), Senna(sennosides A &B), and rhubarb(rhein).

3. Saponin- from colloidal solution that usually foam in water and include Glycyrrhiza(glycyrrhizin) and Dioscorea.

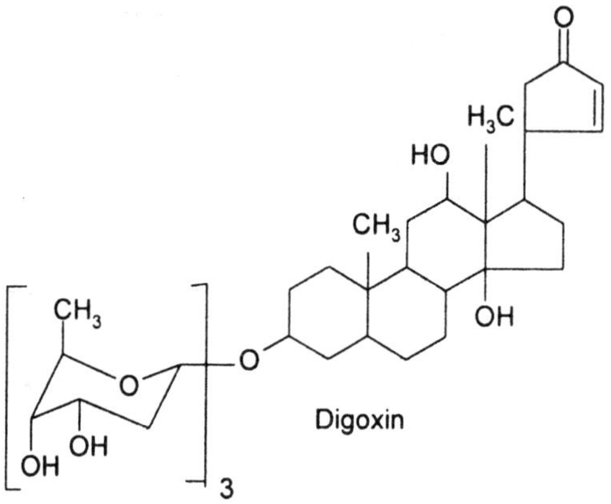

Digoxin

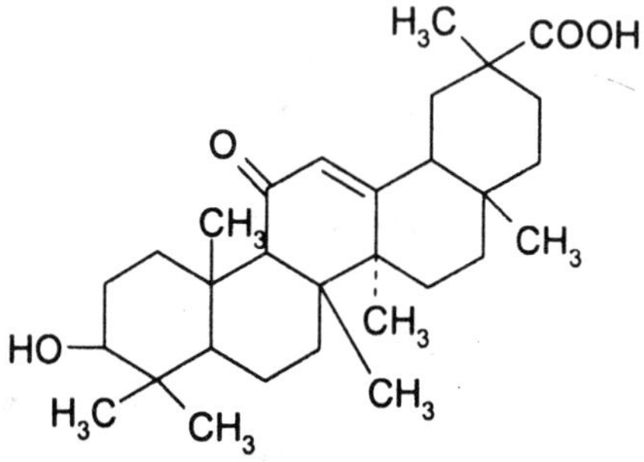

Glycrrhetinic acid(aglycone of glycyrrhizin)

4. Cyanophore-yield hydrocyanic acid as one of the by-product and include Wild cherry(prunasin) and Bitter almond(amygdalin).

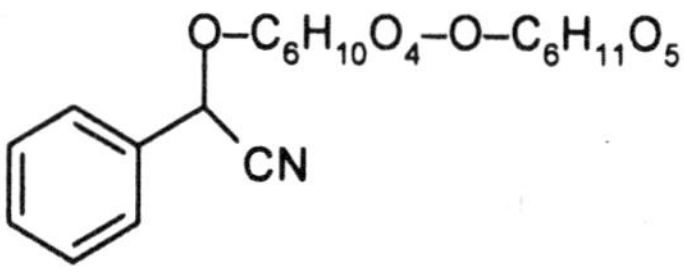

Amygdalin

5. Isothicyanate-when hydrolysed by the enzyme, myrosin yield isothiocyanate as aglycone part and include Black mustard (sinigrin).

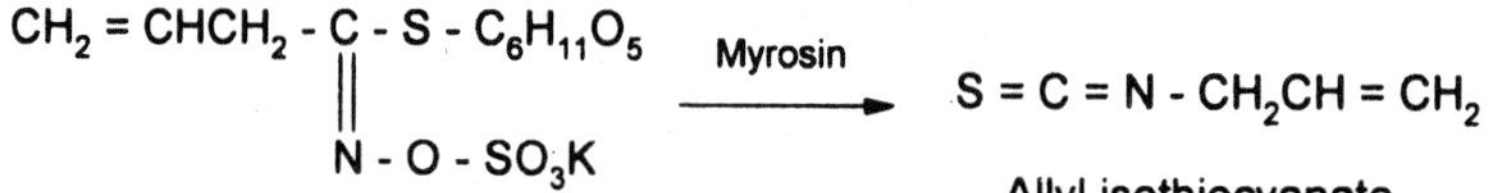

$$CH_2 = CHCH_2 - \underset{\underset{N-O-SO_3K}{\|}}{C} - S - C_6H_{11}O_5 \xrightarrow{\text{Myrosin}} S = C = N - CH_2CH = CH_2$$

Sinigrin

Allyl isothiocyanate

6. Flavonol- include many natural yellow pi gments such as rutin, quercitin and hesperidin

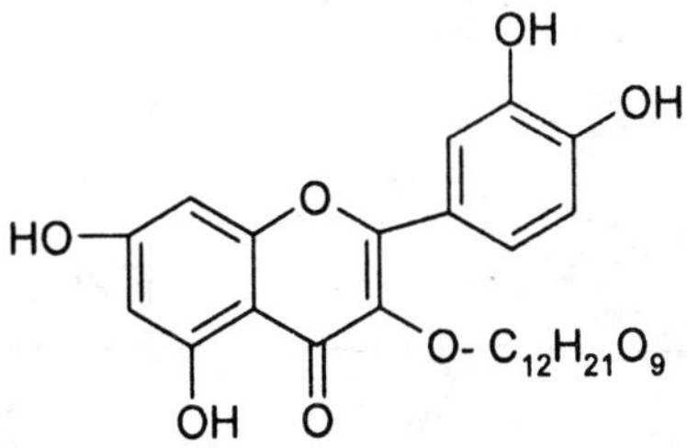

Rutin(Rhamnoglucoside of quercetin)

7. Aldehyde glycosides-have an aldehyde aglycone as chief constituents and include vanillin, used as a flavoring agent.

8. Coumarin glycosides-include Psoralea (psoralen), and Visnega (khellin).

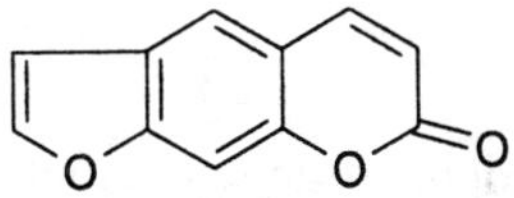

Psoralen

9. Phenol glycosides- contain phenol as aglycone and include bearberry (arbutin).

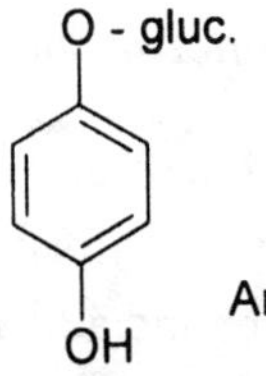

Arbutin

10. Miscellaneous glycosides- Gentiana lutea(gentiopicrin), gymnema(gymnemic acid).

Some color Reactions of Glycosides

Anthraquinone glycosides

Borntrager's test : Extract the powdered drug with ether or any water immiscible organic solvent by heating under refluxing condition and filter. Make alkaline with either caustic soda or ammonia and shake. Observe the resulting coloration in aqueous layer.

Pink, red or violet color appears in aqueous layer. This test is positive with anthraquinone derivatives but negative in case of anthranol(reduced form).

Modified Borntrager's Test : Boil 1 gm of aloe powder with 10 ml of water and filter. Add few drops of ferric chloride solution and dilute hydrochloric acid and shake. Add carbon tetrachloride or ether and shake. Separate out the organic layer and add ammonia solution. Observe the coloration in ammonical layer.

The ammonical layer shows rose-pink to cherry red color, indicating the presence of C-glycosides e.g. aloe-emodin.

Cardiac glycosides

Killer-killiani test : Boil the powdered digitalis about 1 gm with alcohol for 5 minutes and filter. To the filtrate, add 5 ml of water and 0.5 ml of strong solution of lead acetate. Shake well and filter. To the filtrate, add equal volume of chloroform and shake. Separate out the chloroform layer and evaporate to yield the concentrated extract. Dissolve the extract in glacial acetic acid and after cooling add 2 drops of ferric chloride solution. Add concentrated sulphuric acid without disturbing the content in test tube. Observe the change in color at the junction of two layers.

A reddish brown color appears which changes to bluish green after standing for few minutes. This test is positive due to presence of desoxy sugar, digitoxose.

Flavonoidal glycosides

Ammonia Test : Expose a filter paper dipped in an alcoholic solution o the flavonoid to the vapors of ammonia solution. Observe the color on filter paper.

A yellow color appears.

Shinoda Test : To an alcoholic solution of the extract, add few chips of magnesium turnings and dilute HCl solution. Observe the resulting coloration.

A red color is produced.

Vanillin-HCl Test : To the alcoholic solution, add vanillin-HCl reagent. Observe the resulting coloration.

A pink color appears.

The Chemistry and Isolation of Hecogenin from Agave (Sosal Leaves)

The Hecogenin is a Steroidal sapogenin (like diosgenin). It is used in the partial synthesis of cortisones and sex hormones. It is present in Agave sislanes.

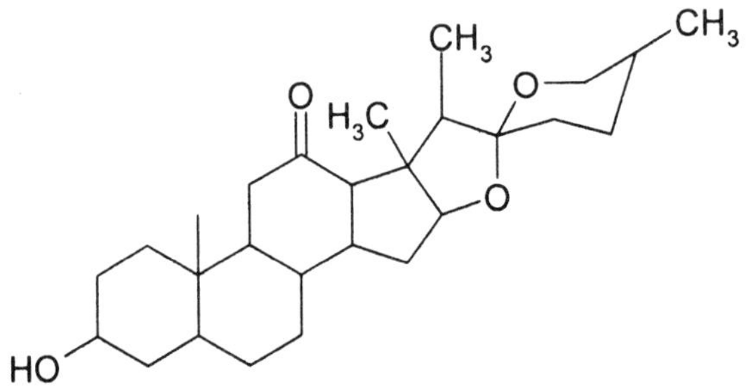

Hecogenin
(O-{0-b-D-glucopyranosyl (1à2)-O-[b-D-xylopyranosyl(1à3)-
O-b-D-glucopyranosyl-(1à4)-b-D-galactopyranoside)

Extraction procedure

(i) Place powdered leaves(1 kg) in a steam-jacketed kettle equipped with an air stirrer. Add Ethanol or isopropanol (4 litres)(85 to 95 per cent) until the plant material is covered by approximately an inch of solvent and then refluxed for 45 minutes with constant stirring. Cool down the suspension and then and filter through a canvas filter. Add second charge of solvent and repeat the process. After the second extraction, allow the residual mass to dry in air overnight and reground to pass through-a 1/16 inch screen. Extract the finely ground material a third time. Combine all the alcoholic extracts and concentrate at atmospheric pressure to 1 litre.

(ii) Extract the concentrated mass with benzene to remove the interfering fat-soluble material

214

and plant pi gments. (The "defatting" is best carried out in a continuous liquid-liquid extractor in order to avoid emulsions).

(iii) After the benzene extraction, wash the benzene layer once with small quantity of 50 per cent ethanol (separatory funnel), and then combine the alcoholic aqueous layer with the main benzene-extracted alcoholic fraction. Discard the benzene layer.

(iv) Concentrate the benzene-extracted aqueous alcohol solution to remove as much alcohol as possible and yet remain free flowing. To the rather turbid aqueous solution, add 5 gm. of sodium chloride per 100 ml. of extract and sufficient HCl to make the pH 4.0 to 5.0. This conditions favor the transfer of saponins into the butanol phase.

(v) Shake the extract thus obtained in separatory funnel four times with butanol saturated with water; 0.5 volume of butanol to 1 volume of extract is used for each extraction. Combine the butanol layers and wash once with 5 per cent aqueous sodium chloride solution. Extract the washings with 0.5 liter of butanol. Then discard the aqueous layers.

(vi) Add the sufficient quantity of water equal to half the volume of butanol to the butanol-saponin extract. Concentrate the two-phase system at atmospheric pressure to a volume. Under these conditions, the butanol is driven off in a constant boiling mixture and can be reused.

(vii) To the aqueous, turbid, saponin solution, add sufficient 95 per cent ethanol so that the final solution is 25 per cent ethanol by volume. Addition of alcohol increases the solubility of the saponins and also reduces foaming during the subsequent hydrolysis step.

(viii) Add sufficient concentrated hydrochloric acid to the aqueous saponin solution to make it 4 N.

(ix) Reflux the solution for 3 to 4 hrs, cool, and filter, and wash the crude, tarry sapogenin precipitate with 50 per cent aqueous ethanol.

(x) Reflux the precipitate for 1 hr with a mixture of benzene and methanol (3:1) containing 200 gm. of potassium hydroxide. Cool down the solution and filter, and any residue is washed with hot benzene containing 10 per cent ethanol. Combine the filtrate and washings, add water, and the aqueous layer is drawn off. The aqueous layer is then twice reextracted with benzene each time. All the benzene solutions are combined and concentrated to dryness to get crude hecogenin.

(xi) Since most sapogenins are quite insoluble in cold acetone, methanol, or hexane, resinous material if present as impurity can be removed by triturating the finely ground crude sapogenin with one of these solvents and filtering. The procedure and solvent vary from sample to sample and must be used with caution. The filtrate should always be evaporated and examined for the presence of appreciable quantities of sapogenins by means of crystallization and chromatography.

(xii) Crystallize the crude hecogenin from ether-methanol, m.p.268°C.

(xiii) Prepare the acetate derivative by refluxing the genins for 1 hr with an excess of acetic anhydride containing a few drops of pyridine. Cool the solution and filter off the genin.

(xiv) Recrystallized from methanol and determine its melting point. It m.p. is 245°C.

The Chemistry and Isolation of Hesperidin

The favonoid compounds can be regarded as C_6-C_3-C_6 compounds, in which each C6 moiety is a benzene ring and the variation in the state of oxidation of the connecting C3 ring determines the properties and class of each compound. Flavonoids occur in all parts of plants, including the fruit, pollen, roots and heartwood. Numerous physiological activities have been attributed to them:

thus, small quantities of flavones may act as cardiac stimulants, others (eg hesperidin (I)), appear to strengthen weak capillary blood vessels, and highly hydroxylated flavones act as antioxidants for fats.

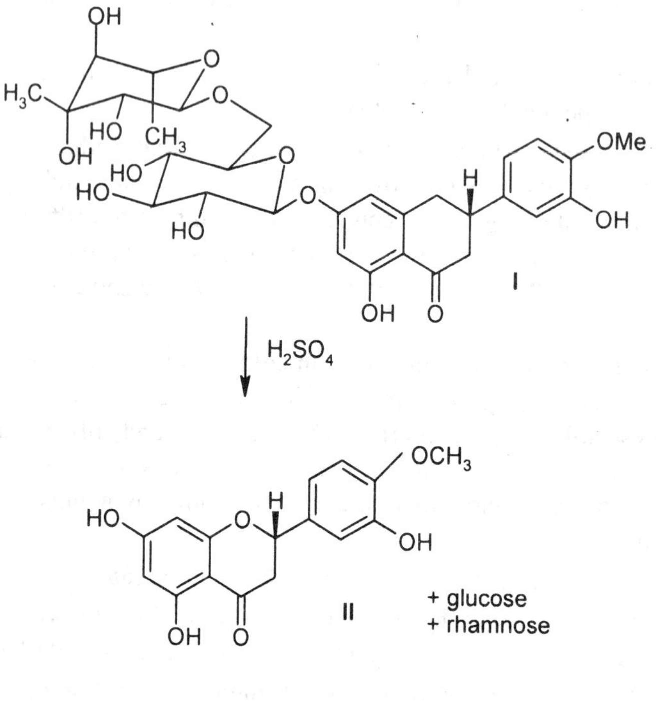

Flavonoid compounds and the related coumarins usually occur in plants as glycosides, in which one or more of the phenolic hydroxyl groups are combined with sugar residues. Acidic degradation of such a glycoside yields an aglycone, e.g. hesperetin (**II**), and the sugars. Hesperidin (**I**) was first isolated in 1828 from the albedo (the spongy inner portion of the peel) of oranges, and has since been found in lemons and other citrus fruits.

This experiment will explore the isolation of the natural product, and some of the differences in chemistry between the glycoside and the aglycone. Hesperetin will also be characterized by several spectroscopic methods.

1. Isolation of Hesperidin (I)

Hesperidin may be extracted from orange peel by the procedure below. It is important to have a good quantity of albedo and *not* just the outer orange coloured part of the peel. For this experiment, you are required to supply your own orange peels (try "Orange Julius" if necessary).

Place powdered dried orange peel (150 gm) and petroleum ether (750 ml) in a round bottomed flask and then heat at reflux for one hr. While hot, filter the mixture through a Buchner funnel. Allow the powder to dry at room temperature and re-extract with refluxing methanol (750 ml) for two hrs. Filter the hot solution and then concentratie the filtrate under reduced pressure to provide a syrup. Crystallize this syrup by the procedure given below.

Recrystallization of Hesperidin (I)

Add the crude hesperidin to dimethylformamide (7 ml per gm of syrup). Stirr the mixture vigorously at room temperature for 15 min, and then filter to remove any insoluble material. To save some time and materials, don't try to recrystallize more than 7.5 gm of the syrup. In a fumehood, add the filtrate dropwise with stirring to a boiling solution of water (20 ml per gm of hesperidin) and acetic acid (0.5 ml per gm of hesperidin). Allow the mixture to cool to get hesperidin.

Collect the precipitated hesperidin by suction filtration and then wash with a little cold water.

Obtain IR and UV spectra of hesperidin and carry out a ferric chloride test. Pure hesperidin has mp 252-254°C.

The compound givesa wine-red colour with alcoholic ferric chloride.

2. Hesperetin (II)1

Stir a mixture of hesperidin (0.7 gm), methanol (25 ml) and concentrated sulphuric acid (0.4 ml) and then heat at reflux overnight. Cool down the resulting homogeneous solution, then concentrate, and finally dilute the residue with ethyl acetate (60 ml). Wash the organic solution with water (3 x20 ml), and the dry with magnesium sulphate. Keep the aqueous washings for an optional analysis of the sugar residues as described below. Concentrate the organic solution to obtain crude hesperetin as a yellow solid. Hesperetin is purified by the following procedure:

Dissolve the crude product in minimum of acetone, and add the resulting solution to a vigorously stirred mixture of water (20 ml) and acetic acid (0.3 ml). Cool the mixture in an ice bath, collect the precipitated hesperetin and wash the crystals with water. Pure hesperetin has mp 220-221°C.

Analysis of the Products

Carry out a ferric chloride test on both **I** and **II**. Explain the differences in terms of the structure of the two materials.

Record the UV spectrum of both **I** and **II** in ethanol. It is not required to know the concentration.

Compare and describe the behaviour of both **I** and **II** towards base by adding a small amount of solid sodium acetate to your UV sample, and recording the new spectrum. Consult the literature and predict the difference in the UV maxima before and after the addition of the base.

Record the IR spectrum of hesperetin as a KBr disk. You may wish to record the IR spectrum of the glycoside as well.

The Chemistry and Isolation of Aloin from Aloe

The most important constituents of Aloes are the two Aloins, Barbaloin and Isobarbaloin, which constitute the so-called 'crystalline' Aloin, present in the drug at from 1O to 30 per cent. Both are C-glycosides of aloe emodin. Other constituents are amorphous Aloin, resin and Aloe-emodin. The proportion in which the Aloins are present in the respective Aloes is not accurately known. The manner in which the evaporation is conducted has a marked effect on the appearance of the Aloes, slow and moderate concentration tending to induce crystallization of the Aloin, thus causing the drug to appear opaque. Such Aloes is termed 'livery' or hepatic, and splinters of it exhibit minute crystals of Aloin when examined under the microscope. If, on the other hand, the evaporation is carried as far as possible, the Aloin does not crystallize and small fra gments of the drug appear transparent; it is then termed 'glassy,' 'vitreous,' or 'lucid' Aloes and exhibits no crystals of Aloin under the microscope.

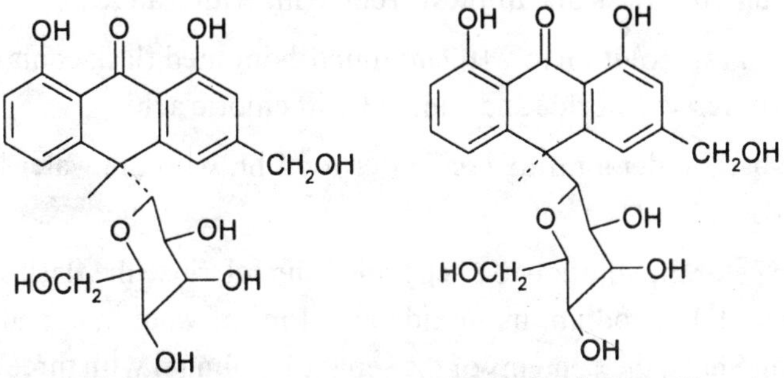

Isobarbaloin(aloin B)   Barbaloin(aloin A)

(10-(1,5-anhydroglucosyl0-aloe-emodin-9-anthrone)

Isolation Procedure

Dissolve powdered aloe (100 gm) in boiling water (1 litre)), stir and filter. Acidify the filtrate with sulphuric acid to precipitate the resinous mass. Separate the precipitate by vacuum filtration and discard. Neutralize the filtrate with ammonia, and allow to stand overnight. Filter the crystalline product and recrystallize from 50% ethanol, yield 10–15%.

Assay of Aloes for Barbaloin Content

Aloe contains hydroxyanthracene derivatives, expressed as barbaloin($C_{21}H_{22}O_9$) and calculated with reference to the dried drug.

Assay procedure

1. Introduce 0.3 gm of powdered drug into 250 ml conical flask. Moisten with 2 ml of methanol, add 5 ml of water warmed to about 60^0C, mix, add a further 75 ml of water at about 60^0C and shake for 30 minutes.

2. Cool, filter into volumetric flask, rinse the conical flask and filter with 20 ml of water, add the rinsing to the volumetric flask and dilute to 1000.0 ml with water.

3. Transfer 10.0 ml of this solution to a 100 ml round-bottomed flask containing 1 ml of a 600 gm/litre solution of ferric chloride and 6 ml of hydrochloric acid.

4. Heat on a water-bath under a reflux condenser for 4 hr, with the water level above that of the liquid in the flask.

5. Allow to cool, transfer the solution to a separating funnel, rinse the flask successively with 4 ml of water, 4 ml of 1M sodium hydroxide and 4 ml of water and add the rinsing to the separating funnel. Shake the contents of the separating funnel with three quantities, each of 20 ml of ether.

6. Wash the combined ether layers with two quantities, each of 10 ml of water.

7. Discard the washings and dilute the organic ohase to 100.0 ml with ether.

8. Evaporate 20.0 ml carefully to dryness on a water-bath and dissolve the residue in 10.0 ml of a 5 gm/litre solution of magnesium acetate in methanol.

*B.P 2005 method

9. Measure the absorbance at 512nm using methanol as compensation liquid.

10. Calculate the %content of hydroxyanthracene derivatives, as barbaloin, from the expression:

$$\frac{A \times 19.6}{m}$$

A = absorbance at 512 nm

m = mass of the substance to be examined in grams

Isolation of Sennosides as Calcium Salts from Senna Leaves

The leaves of *Cassia angustifolia* contain about 2.5% of total sennosides, calculated as sennoside B. These compounds are extracted as their calcium salts from the leaves and pods of Senna.

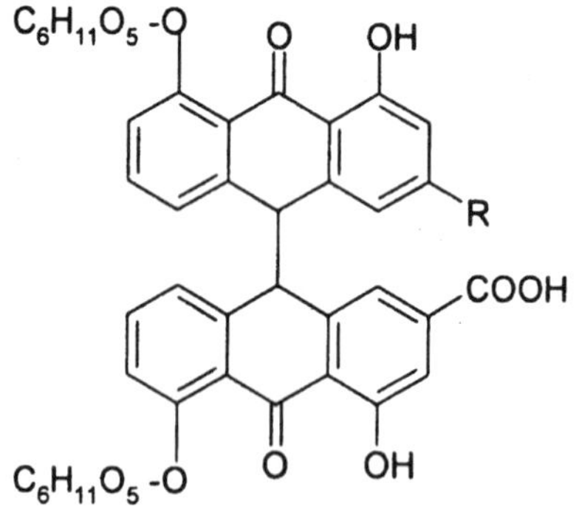

	R	10–10'
Sennoside A	COOH	trans
Sennoside B	COOH	meso
Sennoside C	CH2OH	trans
Sennoside D	CH2OH	meso

Sennosides are hydroxyanthracene O-glycosides derived from Senna leaves. They have been used as natural, safe time-tested laxatives in traditional as well as modern systems of medicine. Available in various convenient dosage forms they can be used to relieve occasional as well as habitual constipation

Procedure

(i) Extract powdered leaves (250 gm) with benzene (750 ml) for 2.5 hrs in a Soxhlet apparatus. Concentrate the extract in vacuum to get a dark green viscous mass.

(ii) Dry the leaves left after benzene extraction in air and re–extract with 70%methanol (750 ml) on a shaker for 6 hrs.

(iii) Filter the extract and extract again the leaves with 70% methanol (500 ml) for 3 hrs. Filter the solvent and combine the methanolic extracts.

(iv) Concentrate the extract to 150 ml and acidify to pH 3.2 with constant stirring.

(v) Cool down the mixture for 2.5 hrs at 5oC, filter in vacuum and add anhydrous calcium chloride (2.5 gm in 35 ml ethanol) to the filter with stirring.

(vi) Adjust pH of the solution to 8 with ammonia solution and set aside for 2.5 hrs.

(vii) Filter the solution in vacuum and dry the precipitate in a desiccator containing phosphorus pentaoxide.

Determination of Sennosides in Senna Leaf

Senna leaf consists of the dried leaflets of *Cassia senna* L. (*C. acutifolia* Delile), known as Alexandrian or Khartoum senna, or *Cassia angustifolia* Vahl, known as Tinnevelly senna, or a mixture of the two species. Acccording to IP, it contains not less than 2.5 % of hydroxyanthracene glycosides, calculated as sennoside B ($C_{42}H_{38}O_{20}$) with reference to the dried drug.

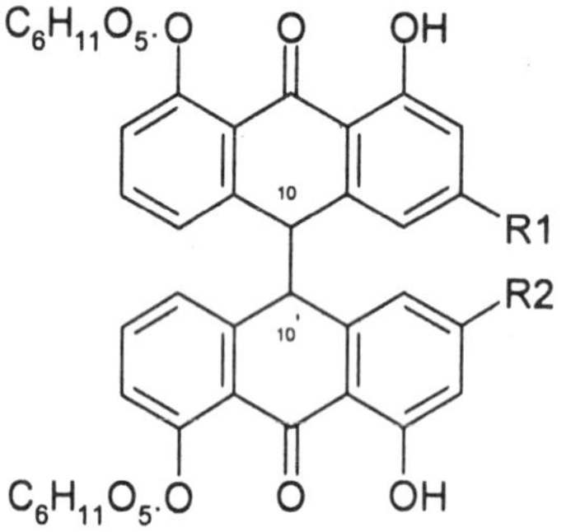

Sennoside A; R_1 = COOH, R_2 = COOH, 10-10' = trans
Sennoside B; R_1 = COOH, R_2 = COOH, 10-10' = meso
Sennoside C; R_1 = CH$_2$OH, R_2 = COOH, 10-10' = trans
Sennoside D; R_1 = CH$_2$OH, R_2 = COOH, 10-10' = meso

Experimental procedure*

1. Place 0.150 gm of the powdered drug in a 100 ml flask. Add 30 ml of water, mix, weigh and place in a water-bath. Heat under a reflux condenser for 15 min.

2. Allow to cool, weigh and adjust to the original mass with water.

---

* B. P. 2005 method

224

3. Centrifuge and transfer 20 ml of the supernatant liquid to a 150 ml separating funnel. Add 0.1 ml of dilute hydrochloric acid and shake with three quantities, each of 15 ml of chloroform.

4. Allow to separate and discard the chloroform layer.

5. Add 0.10 gm of sodium hydrogen carbonate and shake for 3 minutes.

6. Centrifuge and transfer 10 ml of the supernatant liquid to a 100 ml round-bottomed flask with a ground-glass neck.

7. Add 20 ml of ferric chloride solution and mix.

8. Heat for 20 min under a reflux condenser in a water-bath with the water level above that of the liquid in the flask; add 1 ml of hydrochloric acid and heat for a further 20 min, with frequent shaking, to dissolve the precipitate.

9. Cool, transfer the mixture to a separating funnel and shake with three quantities, each of 25 ml, of ether previously used to rinse the flask.

10. Combine the ether layers and wash with two quantities, each of 15 ml, of water. Transfer the ether layers to a volumetric flask and dilute to 100.0 ml with ether.

11. Evaporate 10 ml carefully to dryness and dissolve the residue in 10 ml of a 5 gm/l solution of magnesium acetate in methanol.

12. Measure the extinction immediately of a 1-cm layer of resulting solution at 515 nm, using methanol as the compensation liquid.

13. Calculate the percentage content of sennoside B from the expression:

$$\% \text{ Sennoside content} = \frac{\text{Absorbance at } 515 \text{ nm} \times 1.25}{\text{Mass of drug in gm}}$$

Determination of Cardiac Glycosides in Digitalis Leaves

Digitalis leaf consists of the dried leaf of *Digitalis purpurea* L. It contains not less than 0.3 % of cardenolic glycosides, expressed as digitoxin, and calculated with reference to the drug dried at 100°C to 105°C.

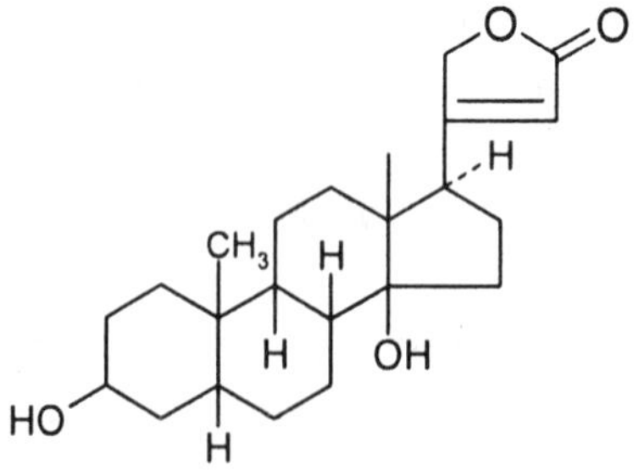

Digitoxigenin

Method 1*

1. Shake 0.250 gm of the powdered drug with 50 ml of water for 1 hr.
2. Add 5 ml of a 150 g/l solution of lead acetate, shake and after a few minutes. Add 7.5 ml of a 40 gm/l solution of disodium hydrogen phosphate.
3. Filter through a pleated filter paper.
4. Heat 50 ml of the filtrate with 5 ml of hydrochloric acid (150 gm/l HCl) under a reflux condenser on a water-bath for 1 hr.
5. Transfer to a separating funnel, rinse the flask with two quantities, each of 5 ml, of water and shake with three quantities, each of 25 ml, of chloroform.
6. Dry the combined chloroform layers over anhydrous sodium sulphate and dilute to 100 ml with chloroform.

---

* B. P. 2005 method

7. Evaporate 40 ml of the chloroformic solution to dryness, dissolve the residue in 7 ml of alcohol (50% V/V) and add 2 ml of dinitrobenzoic acid solution and 1 ml of 1M sodium hydroxide.

8. **Preparation of reference solution:** Dissolve 50 mg of digitoxin in alcohol and dilute to 50 ml with the same solvent. Dilute 5 ml of the solution to 50 ml with alcohol. To 5 ml of the resulting solution add 25 ml of water and 3 ml of hydrochloric acid (150 g ml HCl). Heat the solution under a reflux condenser on a water-bath for 1 hr and complete the preparation as described above.

9. Measure the absorbance of the two solutions at 540 nm several times during the first 12 min until the maximum is reached, using as the compensation liquid a mixture of 7 ml of alcohol (50 % V/V), 2 ml of 3,5-dinitrobenzoic acid solution and 1 ml of 1M sodium hydroxide.

10. From the absorbance measured and the concentrations of the solutions, calculate the content of cardenolic glycosides, expressed as digitoxin.

Method 2*

Digitalis glycosides give an orange red color with Baljet's reagent (picric acid in alkaline medium). This color obeys Beer's law and the intensity of the developed color could be read in a colorimeter at 495 nm. The percentage of glycosides is calculated by referring to a standard curve using the pure glycoside (digitoxin) or by using

$$E_{1\%}^{1\,cm}$$

1. Prepare a 10% tincture of digitalis in alcohol (70%) by maceration of powdered digitalis leaves with alcohol (70%) overnight, then filter.

2. Transfer 8 ml of tincture Digitalis into a 100 ml measuring flask by a graduated pipette.

3. Add 8 ml of 12.5% solution of lead acetate (to precipitate fats, pi gments, resins, tannins and coloring matters). Complete volume by water and mix well. Filter and wash the flask by first 10 ml of the filtrate.

4. Transfer 50 ml of the filtrate into another 100 ml measuring flask by a pipette. Add 8 ml of 12.5% solution of disodium hydrogen phosphate. Mix well and complete to volume using water. Shake well and filter through a filter paper. Wash the filtration flask with the first portion of the filtrate.

5. Transfer 10 ml of the filtrate into a clean test tube. Add 10 ml of freshly prepared Baljet's reagent (9.5 ml of 1% picric acid and 0.5 ml of 5% sodium hydroxide). Set aside for 1 hr(time is necessary for development of the color).

6. Carry out a blank experiment at the same time using 10 ml of water (instead of purified tincture) plus 10 ml Baljet's reagent and set aside for 1 hr.

7. After 1 hr, dilute the solution in each of the experiment and blank with 20 ml of water and mix.

8. Read absorbance of the produced color at 495 nm.

9. The percentage of total glycosides is calculated as digitoxin by referring to the given standard curve or by using the of digitoxin.

$$E_{1\%}^{1\,cm}$$

   a. Standard curve of digitoxin: This can be prepared by using series of dilutions ranging between 50¼g/ ml to 400 ¼g/ ml.

   b. The method by using :

$$E_{1\%}^{1\,cm}$$

As the absorbance of 1 mg digitoxin dissolved in 40 ml final volume (10 ml 70% ethanol plus 10 ml Baljet's reagent and 20 ml water) was found to be 0.425 i.e. that of 2.5 mg/100 ml or 0.0025g/100 ml = 0.425.

Hence that of 1% solution or E1% will be $= \dfrac{0.425}{0.0025} = 170$

Calculation of the results

8 ml of 10% tincture is diluted during purification to 200 ml from which 10 ml are used along with addition of 10 ml Baljet's reagent and 20 ml of water thus making a final volume of 40 ml.

Since 10% tincture i.e. 10 g powder   → made up to 100 ml

                                  X g   → made up to 8 ml

Hence, 8 ml of extract $\equiv [8 \times 10] / 100$

                                        $\equiv 0.8$ gm of powder

and 0.8 g powder $\equiv 200$ ml purified extract.

Amount of powder $\equiv 10$ ml purified extract

                                      $= \dfrac{0.8 \times 10}{200}$

                                        $= 0.04$ gm powder

Absorbance at 1% concentration $= E1\%$

                                        $= 170$

Absorbance at concentration X% $= A$ (measured)

Hence, X $= \dfrac{A}{170}$

i.e. amount of glycosides present in 100 ml solution

Amount present in 1 ml of measured solution $= \dfrac{A}{170 \times 100}$

Amount present in 40 ml measured solution $= \dfrac{A \times 40}{170 \times 100}$

which is also the amount of glycoside present
in 10 ml of the purified tincture

$= 0.04$ g powdered leaves.

Hence, % of glycoside $= \dfrac{A \times 40 \times 100}{170 \times 100 \times 0.04}$

gm of total glycosides calculated as digitoxin $= \dfrac{A \times 100}{17}$

The Chemistry and Isolation of Ammonium Glycyrrhizinate from Liquorice

Licorice root contains from 5 to 10 per cent of its characteristic principle glycyrrhizin; in addition it also contains 5 or 10 per cent of sugars, some bitter substances, beside resins, cellulose, lignin, etc.

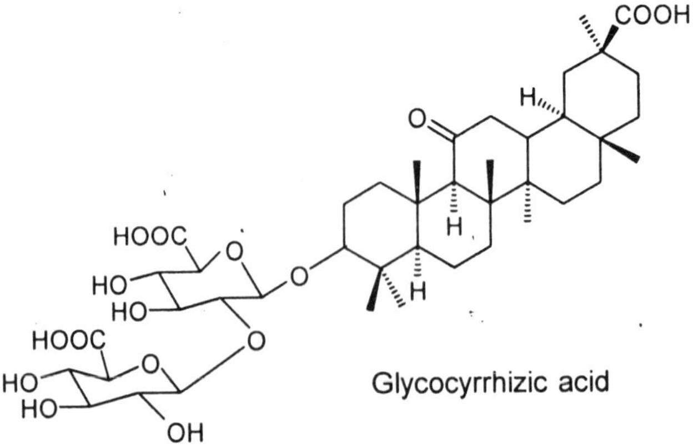

Glycocyrrhizic acid

Glycyrrhizin, a triterpenoid compound, accounts for the sweet taste of licorice root. This compound represents a mixture of potassium-calcium-magnesium salts of glycyrrhizic acid that varies within a 2-25 percent range. Among the natural saponins, glycyrrhizic acid is a molecule composed of a hydrophilic part, two molecules of glucuronic acid, and a hydrophobic fra gment, glycyrrhetic acid.

Glycyrrhizin and other licorice root products have been used for numerous medical purposes, particularly treatment of peptic ulcers and as an expectorant. The triterpene derivative of glycyrrhizin, glycyrrhetinic acid, is itself effective in treatment of peptic ulcer. A synthetic analog, carbenoxolone, was developed in Britain. Both glycyrrhetinic acid and carbenoxolone have a modulatory effect on neural signaling through gap junction channels.

Isolation procedure

1. **Moisten the 500 gm of Glycyrrhiza** powder (No. 20) with the mixture of ammonia water and water (450 ml water and 25 ml of ammonia water) and macerate for 24 hrs.

2. **Pack it** moderately in a conical glass percolator, and gradually pour water upon it until *five hundred cc.* of percolate are obtained.

3. **Add slowly** to the percolate, with constant stirring, so long as a precipitate is produced.

4. **Collect this** on a strainer, wash it with cold Water until the washings no longer have an acid reaction, redissolve it in water with the aid of Ammonia Water, filter, if necessary, and again add Sulphuric Acid so long as a precipitate is produced.

5. **Collect this,** wash it, dissolve it in a sufficient quantity of Ammonia Water previously diluted with an equal volume of water, and spread the clear solution upon plates of glass, so that, when dry, the product(Ammonium Glycyrrhizinate) may be obtained in scales.

Ammonium Glycyrrhizinate occurs in dark brown or brownish-red scales, without odor, and having a very sweet taste. It is freely soluble in water and soluble in alcohol. Its aqueous solution when heated with potassium hydroxide T.S. evolves ammonia.

Estimation of Glycyrrhizic Acid in Liquorice Root

Liquorice root (Glycyrrhiza glabra) contains 7% glycyrrhizin. It is a sweet principle, consisting of calcium and potassium salt of glycyrrhizinic acid.

Procedure

1. Extract about 50 gm of powdered drug with 500 ml of water at 60^0C for about 6 hrs. Adjust the pH to 6.5-7 with dilute ammonia solution and keep aside for few hrs with occasional shaking.

2. Centrifuge the clear extract and evaporate to 75% of its volume under reduced pressure. Then, this acidulated with sufficient sulphuric acid with constant stirring to separate out the precipitate.

3. Fiter the precipitates of crude glycyrrhizinic acid, wash with water, dry and weigh.

4. Calculate the percentage of glycyrrhizinic acid on the basis of air dried drug.

Antibiotics

Contents

Some Color Reactions of Antibiotics

Antibiotics are natural products obtained from the growth of cultures of cultures of bacteria, molds, and soil actinomycetes. They may be defined as chemical substances derived from or produced by living organism, which, in low concentrations, are destructive or inhibitory to microorganisms. In the beginning of antibiotic therapy most antibiotics were obtained from natural processes, but now the majority is produced synthetically, thus paralleling the history of botanical drugs.

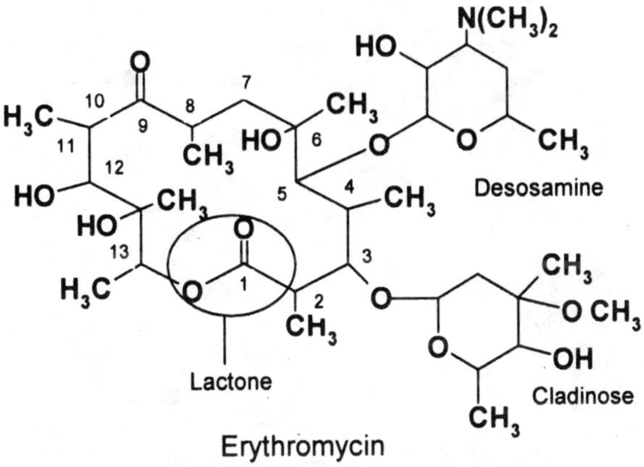

Erythromycin

In this experiment we will test the variant color reactions of three antibiotics(erythromycin, bacitracin, and neomycin sulphate) to common reagents and procedures.

To 5 mg of erythromycin, add 2 ml of dilute H_2SO_4 and shake gently. Repeat this procedure using bacitracin and neomycin sulphate and record the color results.

Result:	Sulphuric acid with Antibiotics
Erthromycin	————
Bacitracin	————
Neomycin sulphate	————

Erthromycin gives reddish brown color. In the neomycin sulphate, there is neither color change nor there is precipitate formation.

To 3 mg of erythromycin add 2 ml of acetone and 2 ml of dilute HCl. Repeat the procedure with bacitracin and neomycin sulphate and record results.

Result:	Hydrochloric acid with Antibiotics
Erthromycin	————
Bacitracin	————
Neomycin sulphate	————

Erthromycin gives purplish-red color. Neomycin sulphate in acidified solution react with few drops of barium chloride gives white precipitate.

To complete this experiment check the microbiological literature and make a list of some of prescription drugs which contain any of these three antibiotics.

Antibacterial Activity of Penicillin G

The earliest antibiotic to be used commercially was penicillin from the Penicillium notatum mold, whose activity was reported by Sir Alexander Flemming in 1929. Tere was now many forms of penicillin employed in medicine today with slightly altered molecular structures.

In this experiment you will be using potassium penicillin G to show its effect on bacterial cultures in broth.

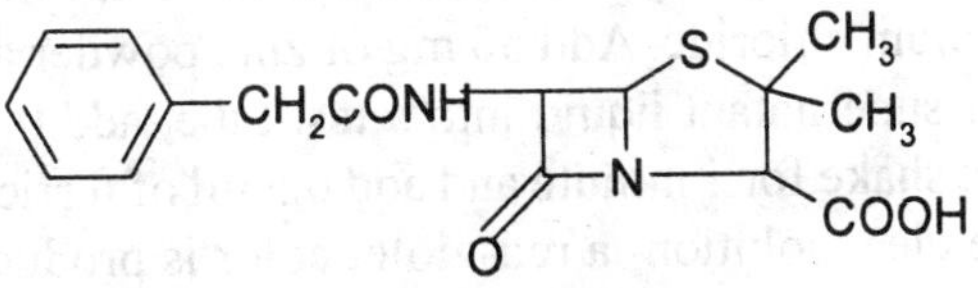

Potassium Penicillin G

To each of four tubes containing 15 ml of fluid thioglycollate medium add 1.0 ml of penicillin solution made to contain 100 USP units of potassium penicillin G in each ml. To each of two of the tubes containing the penicillin broth mixture add sufficient Penicillinase solution(1:10) to inactivate the penicillin. Incubate all four tubes at 37°C for 30minutes, after which time inoculate them with 1.0 ml of a 1:1000 dilution of a culture of Staphylococcus aureus and incubate at 37°C for 24 hrs. For a control, inoculate a tube of medium to which neither penicillin nor Penicillinase has been added. Record results of tubes through 5.

Tube 1. Broth with penicillin & Penicillinase

Tube 2. Broth with penicillin & Penicillinase

Tube 3. Broth with penicillin

Tube 4. Broth with penicillin

Tube 5. Broth with culture only

Assay of Chloramphenicol

Chloramphenicol (chloromycetin) is a white to pale yellow crystalline solid with a bitter taste, moderately toxic to animals and man, particularly to the newborn. Its chief target organ is the blood-forming system. It is an antibiotic produced by Streptomyces venezuelae, and is used in the treatment of Salmonella and otherbacterial infections. It is slightly soluble in water, and freely soluble in alcohol. It is white or slightly yellow needles or plates with a bitter taste.

Identification test : Dissolve 10 mg of of chloramphenico in 1 ml of alcohol(50%) and add 3 ml of 1% w/v solution of calcium chloride. Add 50 mg of zinc powder and heat on a water bath for 10 minutes. Decant the clear supernatant liquid into a test tube, add 0.1 gm of sodium acetate and 2 drops of benzoyl chloride; shake for 1 minute and add 0.5 ml of ferric chloride and if necessary, add sufficient HCl to produce clear solution- a red-violet color is produced. Repeat the test with same quantities of reagents in the same manner but omitting out the zinc powder- no color is produced.

Principle of estimation

Chloramphenicol is reduced in a mixture of glacial acetic acid and water using titanium (III) chloride at room temperature within 10 min. The reduced product was then heated for 20 min with p-dimethylaminobenzaldehyde to yield the final product whose absorbance was used for the determination of the concentration of chloramphenicol. Results obtained with this method were compared with those obtained with the microbiological assay of chloramphenicol.

Chloramphenicol   Chloramphenicol (reduced form)

The final product of the two step reaction was greenish – yellow in colour,, absorbed strongly in the visible region and obeyed Beer's law at $»_{max}$ = 440 nm. The method developed was sensitive and accurately determined chloramphenicol in the presence of common excipients and in different dosage forms.

Chloramphenicol

Dimethylaminobenzaldehyde

Method of estimation

Weigh pure chloramphenicol powder (about 0.1 gm) and transfer into a 20 ml volumetric flask containing a mixture of 3 ml each of glacial acetic acid and distilled water. State the contents of the flask gently to dissolve the powder. Add Titanium (III) chloride (3 ml) mix to the flask and the contents gently. Keep the mixture at room temperature for 10 min to achieve complete reduction of the nitro group of chloramphenicol to a primary aromatic amino group. Pipet out the resulting solution (1 ml) into a 25 ml volumetric flask and make up to volume with methanol. From this solution, 0.2, 0.4, 0.6, 0.8 and 1.0 ml was each pipetted into different 25 ml volumetric flasks. The content of each flask was made up to 1.0 ml by adding 0.8, 0.6, 0.4, 0.2 and 0.0 ml of methanol, respectively. Add the para–dimethylaminobenzaldehyde (10 ml of 0.1% w/v in methanol) to each flask. Mix the contents and heat on a steam bath for 20 min. The flasks were brought out, allowed to cool to room temperature and each made up to volume with methanol. Blank was obtained by repeating the procedure but omitting the drug in the preparations. Time for the completion of each of the two reactions i.e. the reduction and the reaction with para–dimethylaminobenzaldehyde were noted.The wavelength of maximum absorption (lmax) of the product of reaction was also noted.water. The procedure was then continued as for the pure drug above. A Beer's plot was made at the wavelength of maximum absorption from where the concentrations of unknowns were interpolated.

Note : To ensure that the reaction proceeded favourably to the right, the amount of water must be minimised. The initial medium of equal volumes of glacial acetic acid : water (1:1 v/v) has been established to be the optimum condition for aromatic nitro group reduction. Thus by simply mixing chloramphenicol and titanium (III) chloride in the solvent system, the reduction took place easily at room temperature within 10 minutes.

Assay of Benzyl penicillin

Penicillin (sometimes abbreviated **PCN**) is a group of beta-lactam antibiotics used in the treatment of bacterial infections caused by susceptible, usually Gram-positive, organisms. The sodium or potassium salt of benzyl penicillin is colorless or white powder, soluble in water.

Principle of assay

The intact penicillin molecule does not consume iodine while its hydrolytic product, penicilloic acid consumes molecule. The hydrolysis of benzyl penicillin is done by either with alkali or enzyme, lactamase. Hence, intact benzyl penicillin is allowed to react with standard iodine solution. In the same way, the benzyl penicillin after hydrolysis in presence of alkali solution is allowed to react with standard iodine solution. The difference in iodine consumption is analysed for the assay of benzyl penicillin.

Benzyl penicillin

Penicilloic acid

Procedure

Weigh accurately about 60 mg of benzyl penicillin and dissolve in sufficient water to produce 50 ml, transfer 10 ml of the solution to a stoppered flask, add 5 ml of 1N NaOH solution and heat in a water bath for 30 minutes. Add 5.5 ml of 1N HCl solution and 30 ml of of 0.02N iodine, close the flask with a wet stopper, heat in a water bath for 30 minutes, and titrate the excess of iodine with 0.02N sodium thiosulphate, using starch mucilage added toward the end of titration, as indicator. To a further 10 ml of solution of benzyl penicillin prepared in the beginning add 30 ml of 0.02N iodine, and titrate immediately with 0.02N sodium thiosulphate, using starch mucilage added toward the end of titration, as indicator. The difference between the two titrations represent the amount of iodine that is equivalent to the penicillin present.

Each ml of 0.02N iodine = 0.000764 gm of total penicillins, calculated as $C_{16}H_{17}O_4N_2SNa$ or to 0.000798 gm of total penicillins calculated as $C_{16}H_{17}O_4N_2SK$.

Repeat the assay using the standard preparation of penicillin to determine the exact equivalent ml of 0.02N iodine and from this calculate the result of assay.

Natural Colorants

Contents

Introduction to Natural Colorants

The coloring agents are added to :

- Offsetting color loss due to light, air, extremes of temperature, moisture, and storage conditions.
- Masking natural variations in color.
- Enhancing naturally occurring colors.
- Providing identity to foods.
- Protecting flavors and vitamins from damage by light.
- Decorating purposes such as cake icing
- Attract the customers

The coloring agents can be catgorised into natural colorants and synthetic dyes. Natural colorants (to which , you are concerned)can be classified as:-

1. Natural Inorganic Colorants

Inorganic colorants are composed of insoluble metallic compounds which are either derived from natural sources (e.g. china clay, ferric oxide , titanium oxide) or are synthesized. Inorganic colors do not have the same kinds of health risks as organic colors and, therefore do not require certification. Unfortunately, inorganic colorants are not available in the range of shades that the organic offers, and they are not water soluble which limits their range of applications.

Natural Colorants of plant origin

In addition to the inorganic colors, there are other colorants that may be used in cosmetics that are exempt from certification. The typically natural materials like:

Caramel coloring and Carrot oil

Beet extract

Henna

Fruit(citrus, black grapes) & vegetable(reddish, red cabbage, black carrot) juices

Turmeric

Saffron

Indigo

Annato seed

There is no risk in using natural colorant of plant origin but there is no uniformity in coloration. This is the reason of their replacement by synthetic dyes. However, there is question mark on the safety of synthetic dyes.

Natural Colorants of animal origin

Cochineal is coloring agent of animal origin, obtained from larvae of *Coccus cacti*. It is red in color in water and yellow to violet color due to presence of carminic acid.

Isolation of a Carotenoid Pigment :
Bixin from Bixa orellana (Annatto Seeds)

Natural bixin or labile bixin is a polyene in which one double bond has the cis configuration. It is a non-toxic, fat soluble pigment and is, therefore, used as a food coloring agent.

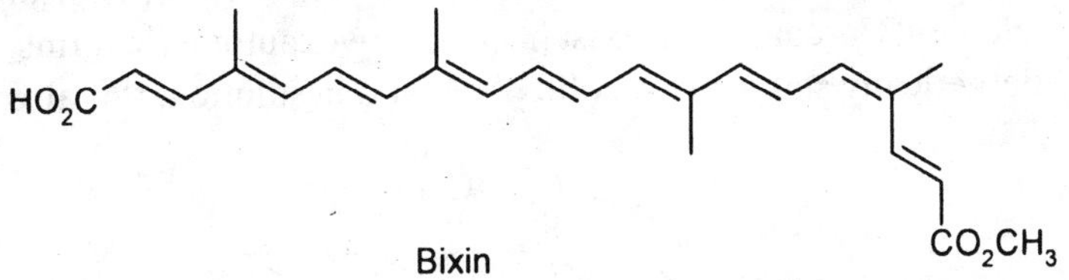

Bixin

Isolation procedure

1. Boil whole seeds of Bixa orellana (do not powder!) with ethyl acetate.
2. Decant the extract and concentrate it to less than half its volume.
3. Collect the pure crystalline bixin which separates out on cooling the concentrated extract on a Büchner funnel.

The average yield is 1.1 gm from 100 gm of the seed. Pour the filtrate into light petrol when a deep-red coloured solid separates out. This is impure bixin. Purer bixin can be obtained by redissolving it in a minimum quantity of ethyl acetate and precipitating it by careful addition of light petrol. By this method another 0.7 to 0.8 gm of pure bixin can be obtained. Pure bixin separates out from ethyl acetate – light petrol as deep red needles.

It gives a blue colour with concentrated sulfuric acid. Its purity can be checked by TLC on silica gel using chloroform-methanol (94:6) as the developing solvent.

Isolation of Curcumin from Turmeric

Curcumin is the principal curcuminoid of the Indian curry spice turmeric, the other two curcuminoids being CurcuminII(demethoxycurcumin) and CurcuminIII(Bis-demethoxycurcumin).The curcuminoids are polyphenols and are responsible for the yellow color of turmeric. It is insoluble in cold water, ether and soluble in alcohol. Curcumin can exist in at least two tautomeric forms, keto and enol. The enol form is more energetically stable in the solid phase and in solution. It is also hepatoprotective.

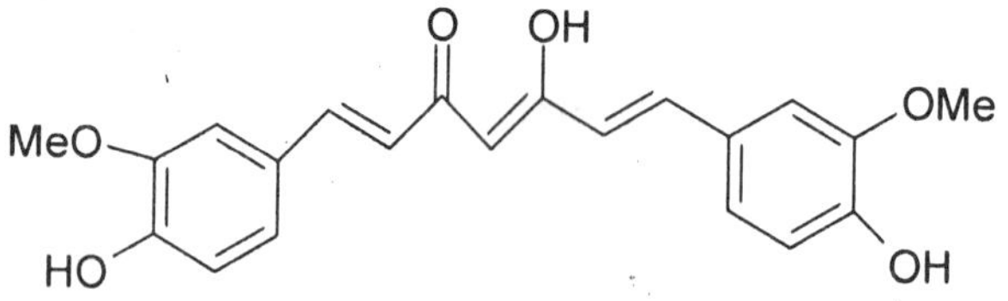

Curcumin

Curcumin can be used for boron quantification in the so-called curcumin method. It reacts with boric acid forming a red colored compound, known as rosocyanine.Since curcumin is brightly colored, it may be used as a food coloring. As a food additive, its E number is E100.

Extraction /isolation of curcuminoids

1. Extract"turmeric powder successively with 95% ethanol at room temperature.
2. Then precipitate with petroleum ether to yield crude curcumin mixture consisted of 78% curcumin I, 16% curcumin II, and 5% curcumin III.
3. Fractionate the crude mixture by silica gel 60 column chromatography using first CHCl3 and then CHCl3/methanol with increasing polarity to isolate pure fractions of curcumins I, II, and III.
4. The identity and purity of each curcuminoids were verified using by TLC, HPLC, IR, MS, and NMR analysis.

Determination of Curcumin Content

Apparatus

(1) Extraction Flask – Flat bottom, 100 ml with TS 24/40 ground glass joint

(2) Condenser – water cooled, drip tip 300-400 mm length TS24/40 ground glass joint

(3) Volumetric Flasks – 100 and 250 ml

(4) Spectrophotometer – any suitable type capable of measuring absorbance at 425 nm

Reagents

(1) Ethyl Alcohol – 95 %

(2) Standard Curcumin solution – weigh 25 mg of standard curcumin into a 100 ml volumetric flask. Dissolve and dilute to mark with alcohol.

Transfer 1 ml of the solution to a 100 ml volumetric flask and dilute to mark with alcohol, This standard solution contains 2 .5 m gm (0.0025 gm) / litre

Procedure

Grind sample as quickly as possible in a grinding mill to pass sieve with 1mm diameter aperture. Weigh accurately about 0.1 gm, add 30 ml alcohol and reflux for two and half hour. Cool the extract and filter quantitatively into a 100 ml volumetric flask Transfer the extracted residue to the filter. Wash thoroughly and dilute to mark with alcohol. Pipette 20 ml of the filtered extract into a 250 ml volumetric flask and dilute to volume with alcohol. Measure the absorbance of the extract and the standard solution at 425 nm in 1 cm cell against an alcohol blank

Calculation

$$\text{Absorptivity of Curcumin, A} = \frac{a\,l}{L \times c} \text{ and}$$

$$\text{Curcumin in Turmeric (\%)} = \frac{a\,2 \times 125 \times 100}{L \times A \times m}$$

where a 1 = absorbance of standard solution at 425 nm

a 2 = absorbance of extract at 425 nm

L = cell length in cm

c = concentration in gm / litre

m = mass in gm of sample

Isolation of Lawsone from Henna leaves

Lawsone (**2-hydroxy-1,4-naphthoquinone**), also known as **hennotannic acid**, is a red-orange dye present in the leaves of the henna plant as well as *Impatiens balsamica* (jewelweed). Humans have used henna extracts containing lawsone as hair and skin pi gments for more than 5000 years. In an acidic solution, lawsone can react via Michael addition with the protein keratin in skin and hair, resulting in a strong permanent stain that lasts until the skin or hair is shed. Lawsone strongly absorbs UV light, and aqueous extracts can be effective, sunless tanning sunscreens.

Lawsone

Isolation procedure

1. Extract the crushed 50 gm fresh leaves of henna by agitation for 2hrs with 250 ml of 20% $NaHCO_3$ soluton.
2. Filter and extract the marc with 100 ml of same solution.
3. Combine the alkaline extract and acidify with dilute sulphuric acid and allow to stand for some time.
4. Filter the crude pruct and re-extract with sufficient quantity of ammonium hydroxide solution and again acidify with dilute HCl solution.
5. Extract the crude product with two times with 50 ml of benzene and filter.
6. Distil out the benzene to get brown colored crystal of Lawsone.
7. Determine its melting point(m.p. 192-193°C).
8. The yield of the product is nearly 1.5% w/w.

Isolation of Lycopene from Tomatoes

Lycopene is a member of the carotenoid family of chemical substances. Lycopene, similar to other carotenoids, is a natural fat-soluble pi gment (red, in the case of lycopene) found in certain plants and microorganisms, where it serves as an accessory light-gathering pi gment and to protect these organisms against the toxic effects of oxygen and light. Thus, Lycopene is a powerfull antioxidant and may also protect humans against certain disorders, such as prostate cancer and perhaps some other cancers, and coronary heart disease.

Carotenoids are the principal pi gments responsible for the red color of red tomatoes. In addition to tomatoes (Lycopersicon esculentum) and tomato-based products, such as ketchup, pizza sauce, tomato juice and tomato paste, lycopene is also found in watermelon, papaya, pink grapefruit and pink guava.

Lycopene is an acyclic isomer of Beta-Carotene. Beta Carotene, which contains beta-ionone rings at each end of the molecule, is formed in plants, including tomatoes, via the action of the enzyme lycopene beta cyclase. Lycopene is a 40 carbon atom, open chain polyisoprenoid with 11 conjugated double bonds. The structural formula of lycopene is represented as follows:

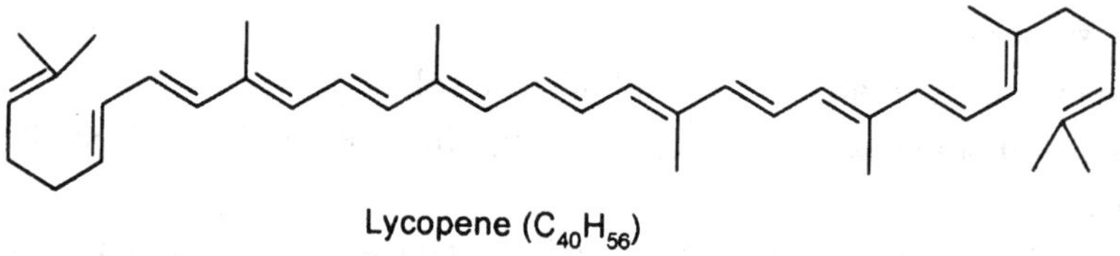

Lycopene ($C_{40}H_{56}$)

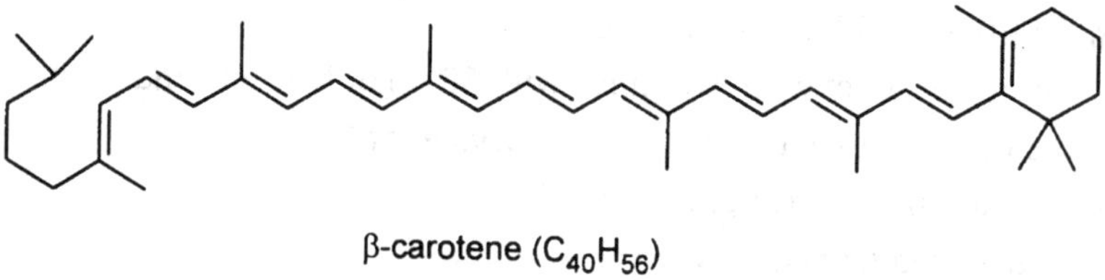

β-carotene ($C_{40}H_{56}$)

Isolation procedure

The two pigments (lycopene and beta carotene) are extracted from tomato paste using a 50:50 hexane-acetone solution and washed with sodium chloride and potassium carbonate. Lycopene was separated from beta carotene through column chromatography. It allows the separation of these pi gments in solution by taking advantage of the varying solubilities and polarities of the dissolved components. In this case, alumina is used as the stationary phase in the column, and hexane was used as the mobile phase to saturate the column and move the components through. Two pi gments, carotene and lycopene, were present in tomato paste in sufficient quantities to observe in the column.

Carotene, with its lesser affinity for alumina, moves through the column first, while lycopene follows shortly after, aided by the addition of acetone.

Spectral analysis of the lycopene reveals that 58% (class results ranged from 28%-63%) of the lycopene is all trans.

1. For "Extraction of Pigments from Tomato Paste," weigh about 1 gm of tomato paste (each section will use a different brand and we'll compare results) into a screwcapvial.

2. Add about 5 ml of 50:50 hexane-acetone solution, cap, and shake vigorously. Let the sediments settle (no need to centrifuge), then use a disposable pipet to remove the liquid portion. Filter the liquid into a collection flask. Repeat this process 4 or 5 times, combining the colored liquid in the same collection flask.

3. Transfer the liquid to a separatory funnel and wash with with saturated NaCl solution, then with 10% K_2CO_3, and finally again with NaCl). Save the organic (top) portion each time, and after the final washing, transfer the organic portion to a beaker and dry it with anhydrous Na_2SO_4.

4. Decant the dried organic phase and evaporate the solution to dryness under vacuum(the air-hose evaporating technique to remove most of the solvent). Save small amount of crude extract for TLC analysis. *(Note: because lycopene is light and sensitive, prevent any unnecessary exposure to light and heat)*.

5. While the solvent is evaporating, set up your chromatography column using neutral alumina in hexane. Gather your organic solution, hexane (the first eluent), 10:90 (% volume) acetone:hexane (the second eluent), a small Erlenmeyer flask,(for collecting the lycopene fraction), and a beaker before you start running your column. By now most of the solvent has evaporated from your sample, and your column is ready to be loaded.

6. If necessary, add a little hexane (1 ml or so) to your sample so that you can transfer it carefully to the top of the column using a pipet.

7. Let the sample load onto the column, then elute with hexane (do NOT let the column go dry). Collect the eluant in a series of test tubes. You should be able to see the bands of pi gment separate on your column; first a thin yellow band (carotene), then a reddish-orange band (lycopene).

8. When the carotene has completely eluted from the column, you can switch to a 10% solution of acetone in hexane to elute the lycopene. You may discard the carotene, but save the

lycopene for UV analysis. Take a TLC of your crude and purified products. Use 10:90 acetone:hexane as the developing solution.

9. You can calculate the % *trans*-lycopene in your section's combined sample from the UV spectrum provided using the empirical method described below. This convention expresses the height of the peak of longest wavelength as a percentage of the height of the peak of maximum absorption, with the baseline being the valley between the two maxima.

· Draw a straight, horizontal line tangent to the bottom of the valley between the last (highest wavelength) two peaks on the spectrum.

· Measure the height of both peaks from that line, calling the heights a and b, respectively.

· Divide the smaller height (b) by the larger (a) and multiply by 100:

(b/a) x 100% = % *trans*-lycopene

Isolation of Chlorophyll and Carotenoid Pigments from Spinach

Carotenoids are part of a larger collection of plant derived compounds called terpenes. These naturally occurring compounds contain 10, 15, 20, 25, 30 and 40 carbon atoms which suggest that there is a compound with five carbon atoms that serves as their building block. Their structures are consistent with the assumption that they were made by joining together isoprene units, usually in a "head to tail" fashion. Isoprene is the common name for 2-methyl-1,3-butadiene. The branched end is the "head" and the unbranched is the "tail". That isoprene units are linked in a head to tail fashion to form terpenes is known as the isoprene rule. Carotenoids are tetraterpenes (eight isoprene units). Lycopene, the compound responsible for the red coloring of tomatoes and watermelon, and β-carotene, the compound that causes carrots and apricots to be orange, are examples of carotenoids.

β-Carotene is also the coloring agent used in margarine. When ingested bð -Carotene is cleaved to form two molecules of vitamin A and is the major dietary source of the vitamin. Vitamin A, also called retinol, plays an important role in vision.

Spinach leaves contain chlorophyll a and b and bð -carotene as major pigments as well as smaller amounts of other pi gments such as xanthophylls which are oxidized versions of carotenes and pheophytins which look like chlorophyll except that the magnesium ion mg^{++} has been replaced by two hydrogen ions $2H^+$. In this experiment, you will isolate and separate the spinach pi gments using differences in polarity to effect the separation. Since the different components are colored differently, you can follow this separation visually. The structures of the major components are given below. Notice that since bð -carotene is a hydrocarbon it is very nonpolar. Both chlorophylls contain C—O and C—N bonds which are polar and also contain magnesium bonded to nitrogen which is such a polar bond it is almost ionic. Both chlorophylls are much more polar than bð -carotene. If you look carefully you can see that the two chlorophylls differ only in one spot. Chlorophyll a has a methyl group (—CH$_3$) in a position where chlorophyll b has an aldehyde (—CHO). This makes chlorophyll b slightly more polar than chlorophyll a. After you isolate the pi gment mixture from the leaves in a hexane solution you will use the difference in polarity to separate the various pi gments using column chromatography. You will also analyze the original extract and the pi gment fractions using thin layer chromatography, which also separates based on polarity.

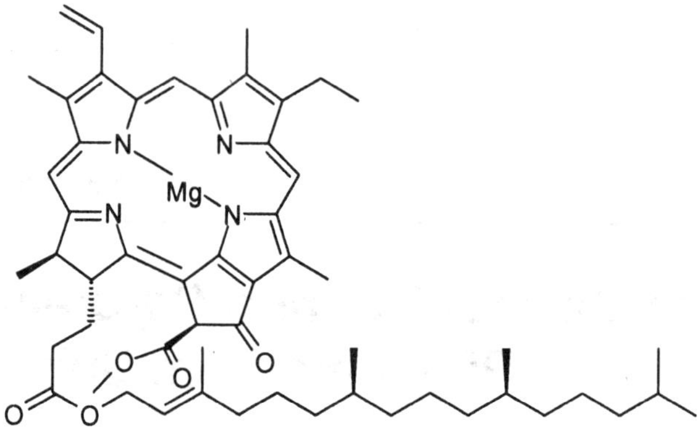

Chlorophyll a (Blue-green, polar)

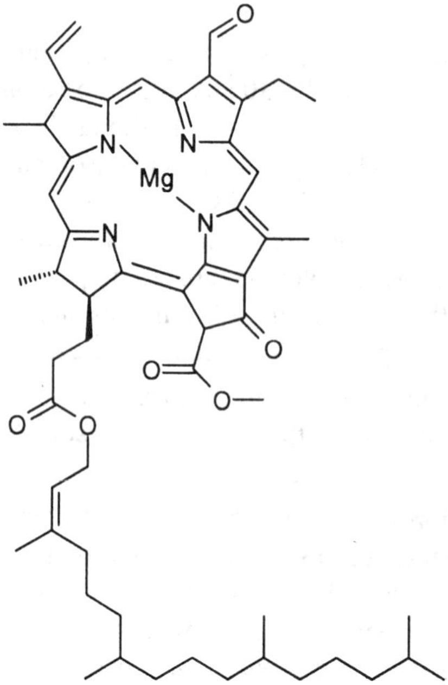

Chlorophyll b (Green, polar)

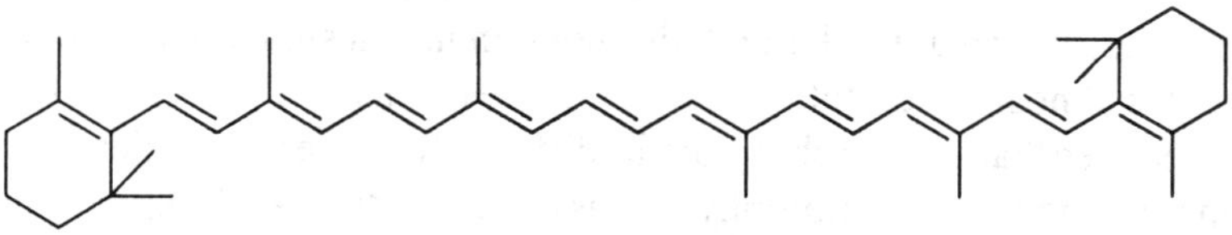

beta-Carotene (yellow, non-polar)

Isolation of pi gment from leaves

1. Weigh about 1.0 gm of fresh spinach leaves (or other fresh green leaves; avoid using stems or thick veins). Place them in a mortar along with 1.0 g of anhydrous magnesium sulphate

and 2.0 gm of sand. Grind with a pestle until a light green power is obtained (about 5-10 minutes).

2. Transfer the mixture to a centrifuge tube. Add 2.0 ml of acetone. Rinse the mortar and pestle with another 2.0 ml of acetone, and transfer the remaining mixture to the centrifuge tube. Cap and shake the mixture and then allow it to stand for 10 minutes. Using a Pasteur pipette, or by careful pouring, transfer the liquid to a vial. Label the vial E for extract. *If time is short, label the vial with your name and store it open in your desk until the next laboratory period.* If there is time to continue the experiment the same day, use a gentle stream of air or nitrogen in the hood to effect a quicker evaporation.

3. Set a Column of Silica gel or Floracil for Column Chromatography of Spinach Pigments in · hexane. Then, arrange the following solvents to your work space before you proceed: hexane, 70% hexane-30% acetone solution (by volume), acetone. You should also have several vials labeled 1, 2, 3, etc., as well as a beaker to hold waste chromatography solvent. Once the procedure is started, it should not be stopped: the florisil must be kept wet with solvent all the time.

4. If your extract vial has dried out, reconstitute it by adding about 1/2 ml of hexane. Set aside about 1/4 of your extract (from vial E) to use for later thin layer chromatography. When you are ready to begin the column chromatography, place the waste solvent beaker under the Pasteur pipette and add about 3.0 ml of hexane to the top of the pipette. As the florisil or silica gel is wetted, the hexane will flow into the beaker. As soon as the solvent is drained so that the top layer of sand is just covered by the solvent, start adding your spinach extract to the top of the column. As the extract drains onto the florisil or silica gel, the pigments will begin to separate with the yellow carotene band getting ahead of the green chlorophyll band. Continue collecting solvent in your waste solvent beaker until the yellow band has reached the bottom of the column and the solvent draining out begins to turn yellow. This yellow band is sometimes very narrow—don't miss it! If 5 ml of hexane is not sufficient to move the yellow band to the bottom of the column, or you don't see a yellow band, add the 90% hexane-10% acetone as needed to move the yellow band out. When the drops are yellow replace the waste beaker with vial #1 and continue collecting in this vial until the drops lose their color or the vial is full. If the yellow band is not finished when the vial is full, continue to collect the yellow band in vial #2, 3, etc. When the yellow band is out of the column, collect any clear solvent in your waste beaker.

When the yellow band is out and the solvent you have most recently added has drained to the top of the sand, add your 70/30 mixture of hexane and acetone to move the green band further down the column. Continue to add this solvent mixture until all 10 ml have been added. Whenever the green color reaches the bottom of the column, remove your waste beaker and put in your next vial and subsequent vials as needed as you continue collecting the green band. When your green band first begins to collect, it may be quite pale. When all 10 ml of the 70/30 mixture have been added, you may need to add the straight acetone to further increase the polarity of the eluting solvent and bring out more of the chlorophyll band. When the major portion of the green band has been collected, replace the latest vial with your waste solvent beaker and allow the residual solvent to drain out of the pipette. *This is another possible stopping point in the experiment.*

5. Before thin layer chromatography (TLC), concentrate your colored solutions so that they will show up better on the TLC plates. A gentle stream of air in a hood is used to evaporate solvent so that only about 1/4 ml of yellow and 1/4 ml of green solution are left. If necessary, combine the contents of your vials as you evaporate so that you end up with just one vial of yellow carotenes and one vial of green chlorophylls. Also evaporate the original extract you saved for TLC so that no more than 1/4 ml is left.

   Perform the TLC of all the fractions as well as of crude extract using developing solvent (70% hexane-30% acetone). After developing, Visible spots should be circled in pencil since the colors may fade over time.

6. Calculate R_f values for each *spot* on your plate. Spots with the same R_f values within experimental error and the same appearance should be the same compound.

   In the crude extract, you may be able to see the following components (in order of decreasing R_f values):

   Carotenes (1 spot) (yellow-orange)

   Pheophytin a (gray, may be nearly as intense as chlorophyll b)

   Pheophytin b (gray, may not be visible)

   Chlorophyll a (blue-green, more intense than chlorophyll b)

   Chlorophyll b (green)

   Xanthophylls (possibly 3 spots: yellow)

Reagents and Solutions

Dilute Acids

Acetic acid, 3 N. Use 172 ml of 17.4 M acid (99-100%). Dilute to one liter.

Hydrochloric acid, 3 N. Use 258 ml of 11.6 M acid (36% HCl). Dilute to one liter.

Nitric acid, 3 N. Use 195 ml of 15.4 M acid (69% HNO_3). Dilute to one liter.

Phosphoric acid, 9 N. Use 205 ml of 14.6 M acid (85% H_3PO_4). Dilute to one liter.

Sulphuric acid, 6 N. Use 168 ml of 17.8 M acid (95% H_2SO_4). Dilute to one liter.

Dilute Bases

Ammonium hydroxide, 3 M, 3 N. Dilute 200 ml of concentrated solution (14.8 M, 28% NH_3) to 1 liter.

Barium hydroxide, 0.2 M, 0.4 N. Saturated solution, 63 gm per liter of $Ba(OH)_2.8H_2O$. Use some excess, filter off $BaCO_3$ and protect from CO_2 of the air with soda lime or ascarite in a guard tube.

Calcium hydroxide, 0.02 M, 0.04 N. Saturated solution, 1.5 gm per liter of $Ca(OH)_2$. Use some excess, filter off $CaCO_3$ and protect from CO_2 of the air.

Potassium hydroxide, 3 M, 3 N. Dissolve 176 gm of the sticks (95%) in water and dilute to 1 liter.

Sodium hydroxide, 1 M, 1 N. Dissolve 39.989 gm of the pure powder (99.9%) in water and dilute to 1 liter.

Sodium hydroxide, 3 M, 3 N. Dissolve 126 gm of the sticks (95%) in water and dilute to 1 liter.

General Reagents

Aluminum chloride, 0.167 M, dissolve 22 gm of $AlCl_3$ in 1 liter of water.

Ammonium acetate, 3 M, 3 N. Dissolve 230 gm of $NH_4C_2H_2O_2$ in water and dilute to 1 liter.

Ammonium carbonate, 1.5 M. Dissolve 144 gm of the commercial salt (mixture of $(NH_4)_2CO_3.H_2O$ and $NH_4CO_2NH_2$) in 500 ml of 3 N NH_4OH and dilute to 1 liter.

Ammonium chloride, 3 M, 3 N. Dissolve 160 gm of NH_4Cl in water. Dilute to 1 liter.

Ammonium molybdate :

1. 0.5 M, 1 N. Mix well 72g of pure MoO_5 (or 81 gm of H_2MoO_4) with 200 ml of water, and add 60 ml of conc. ammonium hydroxide. When solution is complete, filter and pour filtrate, very slowly and with rapid stirring, into a mixture of 270 ml of conc. HNO_3 and 400 ml of water. Allow to stand over night, filter and dilute to 1 liter.

2. The reagent is prepared as two solutions which are mixed as needed, thus always providing fresh reagent of proper strength and composition. Since ammonium molybdate is an expensive reagent, and since an acid solution of this reagent as usually prepared keeps for only a few days, the method proposed will avoid loss of reagent and provide more certain results for quantitative work.

Solution 1: Dissolve 100 gm of ammonium molybdate (C.P. grade) in 400 ml of water and 80 ml of 15 M NH_4OH. Filter if necessary, though this seldom has to be done

Solution 2: Mix 400 ml of 16 M nitric acid with 600 ml of water.

For use, mix the calculated amount of solution 1 with twice its volume of solution 2, adding solution 1 to solution 2 slowly with vigorous stirring. Thus, for amounts of phosphorus up to 20 mg, 10 ml of solution 1 to 20 ml of solution 2 is adequate. Increase amount as needed.

Ammonium nitrate, 1 M, 1 N. Dissolve 80 gm of NH_4NO_3 in 1 liter of water.

Ammonium oxalate, 0.25 M, 0.5 N. Dissolve 35.5 gm of $(NH_4)_2C_2O_4.H_2O$ in water. Dilute to 1 liter.

Ammonium sulphate, 0.25 M, 0,5 N. Dissolve 33 gm of $(NH_4)_2SO_4$ in 1 liter of water.

Ammonium sulphide, colorless:

1. 3 M. Treat 200 ml of conc. NH_4OH with H_2S until saturated, keeping the solution cold. Add 200 ml of conc. NH_4OH and dilute of 1 liter.

2. 6 N. Saturate 6 N ammonium hydroxide (40 ml conc. ammonia solution +60 ml H_2O) with washed H_2S gas. The ammonium hydroxide bottle must be completely full and must be kept surrounded by ice while being saturated (about 48 hours for two liters). The reagent is best preserved in brown, completely filled, glas-stoppered bottles.

Ammonium sulphide, *yellow* : Treat 150 ml of conc. NH_4OH with H_2S until saturated, keeping the solution cool. Add 250 ml of conc. NH_4OH and 10 g of powdered sulfur. Shake the mixture until the sulfur is dissolved and dilute to 1 liter with water. In the solution the concentration of $(NH_4)_2S_2$, $(NH_4)_2S$ and NH_4OH are 0.625, 0.4 and 1.5 normal respectively. On standing, the concentration of $(NH4)2S2$ increases and that of $(NH_4)_2S$ and NH_4OH decreases.

Antimony pentachloride, 0.1 M, 0.5 N. Dissolve 30 gm of $SbCl_5$ in 1 liter of water

Antimony trichloride, 0.167 M, 0.5 N. Dissolve 38 gm of $SbCl_3$ in 1 liter of water.

Aqua regia. Mix 1 part concentrated HNO_3 with 4 parts of concentrated HCl. This formula should include one volume of water if the aqua regia is to be stored for any length of time. Without water, objectionable quantities of chlorine and other gases are evolved.

Barium chloride, 0.25 M, 0.5 N. Dissolve 61 gm of $BaCl_2.2H_2O$ in water. Dilute to 1 liter.

Barium hydroxide, 0,1 M, about 0.2 N. Dissolve 32 gm of $Ba(OH)_2.8H_2O$ in 1 liter of water.

Barium nitrate, 0.25 M, 0.5 N. Dissolve 65 gm of $Ba(NO_3)_2$ in 1 liter of water.

Bismuth chloride, 0.167 M, 0.5 N. Dissolve 53 gm of $BiCl_2$ in 1 liter of dilute HCl, Use 1 part HCl to 5 parts water.

Bismuth nitrate, 0.083 M, 0.25 N. Dissolve 40 gm of $Bi(NO_3)_3.5H_2O$ in 1 liter of dilute HNO_3, Use 1 part of HNO_3 to 5 parts of water.

Cadmium chloride, 0,25 M, 0.5 N. Dissolve 46 g of $CdCl_2$ in 1 liter of water.

Cadmium nitrate, 0.25 M, 0.5 N. Dissolve 77 gm of $Cd(NO_3)$ $2.4H_2O$ in 1 liter of water.

Cadmium sulphate, 0.25 M, 0.5 N. Dissolve 70 gm of $CdSO_4. 4H_2O$ in 1 liter of water.

Calcium chloride, 0.25 M, 0.5 N. Dissolve 55 gm of $CaCl_2.6H_20$ in water. Dilute to 1 liter.

Calcium nitrate, 0.25 M, 0.5 N. Dissolve 41 gm of $Ca(NO_3)_2$ in 1 liter of water.

Chloroplatinic acid:

1. 0.0512 M, 0.102 N. Dissolve 26.53g of $H_2PtCl_4.6H_2O$ in water. Dilute to 100 ml. Contains 0.100 gm Pt per ml

2. Make a 10% solution by dissolving 1 gm of $H_2PtCl_6.6H_2O$ in 9 ml of water. Shake thoroughly to insure complete mixing. Keep in a dropping bottle.

Chromic chloride, 0.167 M, 0.5 N. Dissolve 26 gm of $CrCl_3$ in 1 liter of water.

Chromic nitrate, 0.167 M, 0.5 N. Dissolve 40 gm of $Cr(NO_3)_3$ in 1 liter of water.

Chromic sulphate, 0.083 M, 0.5 N. Dissolve 60g of $Cr_2(SO_4)_3.18H_2O$ in 1 liter of water.

Cobaltous nitrate, 0.25 M, 0.5 N. Dissolve 73 gm of $Co(NO_3)_2.6H_2O$ in 1 liter of water.

Cobaltous sulfate, 0.25 M, 0.5 N. Dissolve 70 gm of CoSO4.7H2O in 1 liter of water.

Cupric chloride, 0.25 M, 0.5 N. Dissolve 43 gm of $CuCl_2.2H_2O$ in 1 liter of water.

Cupric nitrate, 0.25 M, 0.5 N. Dissolve 74 gm of $Cu(NO_3)_2. 6H_2O$ in 1 liter of water.

Cupric sulphate, 0.5 M, 1 N. Dissolve 124. gm of $CuSO_4.5H_2O$ in water to which 5 ml of H_2SO_4 has been added. Dilute to 1 liter.

Ferric chloride, 0.5 M, 1.5 N. Dissolve 135.2 gm of $FeCl_3.6H_2O$ in water containing 20 ml of conc. HCl. Dilute to1 liter.

Ferric nitrate, 0.167 M, 0.5 N. Dissolve 67 gm of $Fe(NO_3)_3$ $9H_2O$ in 1 liter of water.

Ferric sulphate, 0.25 M, 0.5 N. Dissolve 140.5 gm of $Fe_3(SO_4)_3.9H_2O$ in water containing 100 ml of conc. H2SO4. Dilute to 1 liter.

Ferrous ammonium sulfate, 0.5 M, 1 N. Dissolve 196 gm of $Fe(NH_4SO_4)_2.6H_2O$ in water containing 10 ml of conc. H_2SO_4. Dilute to 1 liter. Prepare fresh solutions for best results

Ferrous sulphate, 0.5 M, 1 N. Dissolve 139 gm of $FeSO_4.7H_2O$ in water containing 10 ml of conc. H_2SO_4. Dilute to 1 liter. Solution does not keep well.

Lead acetate, 0.5 M, 1 N. Dissolve 190 gm of $Pb(C_2H_3O_2)_2. 3H_2O$ in water. Dilute to 1 liter.

Lead nitrate, 0.25 M, 0.5 N. Dissolve 83 gm of $Pb(NO_2)_2$ in water. Dilute to one liter.

Lime water. See Calcium hydroxide.

Magnesium chloride, 0.25 M, 0.5 N. Dissolve 51 gm of mg $Cl_2.6H_2O$ in 1 liter of water.

Magnesium chloride reagent. Dissolve 50 gm of mg $C_2.6H_2O$ and 100 gm of NH_4Cl in 500 ml of water. Add 10 ml of conc. NH_4OH, allow to stand over night and filter if a precipitate has formed. Make acid to methyl red with if a dilute HCl. Dilute to 1 liter. Solution contains 0.25 M $MgCl_2$ and 2 M NH_4Cl. Solution may also be diluted with 133 ml of conc. NH_4OH and water to make 1 liter. Such a solution will contain 2 M NH_4OH.

Magnesium nitrate, 0.25 M, 0.5 N. Dissolve 64 gm of mg$(NO_2)_2.6H_2O$ in 1 liter of water.

Magnesium sulphate, 0.25 M, 0.5 N. Dissolve 62 gm of $MgSO_4.7H_2O$ in 1 liter of water.

Manganous chloride, 0.25 M, 0.5 N. Dissolve 50 gm of $MnCl_2.4H_2O$ in 1 liter of water.

Manganous nitrate, 0.25 M, 0.5 N. Dissolve 72 gm of $Mn(NO_3)_2.6H_2O$ in 1 liter of water.

Manganous sulphate, 0.25 M, 0.5 N. Dissolve 69 gmof $MnSO_4.7H_2O$ in 1 liter of water.

Mercuric chloride, 0.25 M, 0.5 N. Dissolve 68 gm of $HgCl_2$ in water. Dilute to 1 liter.

Mercuric nitrate, 0.25 M, 0.5 N. Dissolve 81 gm of $Hg(NO_3)_2$ in 1 liter of water.

Mercuric sulphate, 0.25 M, 0.5 N. Dissolve 74 gm of $HgSO_4$ in 1 liter of water.

Mercurous nitrate. Use 1 part $HgNO_3$, 20 parts water and 1 part HNO_3.

Potassium bromide, 0.5 M, 0.5 N. Dissolve 60 gm of KBr in 1 liter of water.

Potassium carbonate, 1.5 M, 3 N. Dissolve 207 gm of K_2CO_3 in 1 liter of water.

Potassium chloride, 0.5 M, 0.5 N. Dissolve 37 gm of KCl in 1 liter of water.

Potassium chromate, 0.25 M, 0.5 N. Dissolve 49 gm of K_2CrO_4 in 1 liter of water.

Potassium cyanide, 0.5 M, 0.5 N. Dissolve 33 gm of KCN in 1 liter of water.

Potassium dichromate, 0.125 M. Dissolve 37 gm of $K_2Cr_2O_7$ in 1 liter of water.

Potassium ferricyanide, 0.167 M, 0.5 N. Dissolve 55 gm of $K_3Fe(CN)_6$ in 1 liter of water.

Potassium ferrocyanide, 0.5 M, 2 N. Dissolve 211 gm of $K_4Fe(CN)_6.3H_2O$ in water. Dilute to 1 liter.

Potassium iodide, 0.5 M, 0.5 N. Dissolve 83 gm of KI in 1 liter of water.

Potassium nitrate, 0.5 M, 0.5 N. Dissolve 51 gm of KNO_3 in 1 liter of water.

Potassium sulphate, 0.25 M, 0.5 N. Dissolve 44 gm of K_2SO_4 in 1 liter of water.

Silver nitrate, 0.1 M, 0.1 N. Dissolve 16.987 gm of $AgNO_3$ in distilled water. Dilute to 1 liter.

Silver nitrate, 0.5 M, 0.5 N. Dissolve 84.935 gm of $AgNO_3$ in distilled water. Dilute to 1 liter.

Silver nitrate, 1 M, 1 N. Dissolve 169.87 gm of $AgNO_3$ in distilled water. Dilute to 1 liter.

Sodium acetate, 3 M, 3 N. Dissolve 408 gm of $NaC_2H_3O_2.3H_2O$ in water. Dilute to 1 liter.

Sodium carbonate, 1.5 M, 3 N. Dissolve 159 gm of Na_2CO_3, or 430 gm of $Na_2CO_3.10H_2O$ in water. Dilute to 1 liter.

Sodium chloride, 0.5 M, 0.5 N. Dissolve 29 gm of NaCl in 1 liter of water.

Sodium cobaltinitrite, 0.08 M *(reagent for potassium)*. Dissolve 25 gm of $NaNO_2$ in 75 ml of water, add 2 ml of glacial acetic acid and then 2.5g of $Co(NO_3) = 6H_2O$. Allow to stand for several days, filter and dilute to 100 ml. Reagent is somewhat unstable.

Sodium hydrogen phosphate, 0.167 M, 0.5 N. Dissolve 60 gm of $Na_2HPO_4.12H_2O$ in 1 liter of water.

Stannic chloride, 0.125 M, 0.5 N. Dissolve 33 gm of $SnCl_4$ in 1 liter of water.

Stannous chloride, 0.5 M, 1 N. Dissolve 113 gm of $SnCl_2.2H_2O$ in 170 ml of conc. HCl, using heat if necessary. Dilute with water to 1 liter. Add a few pieces of tin foil. Prepare solution fresh at frequent intervals.

Stannous chloride *(for Bettendorf test)*. Dissolve 113 gm of $SnCl_2.2H_2O$ in 75 ml of conc. HCl. Add a few pieces of tin foil.

Strontium chloride, 0.25 M, 0.5 N. Dissolve 67 gm of $SrCl_2.6H_2O$ in 1 liter of water.

Zinc nitrate, 0.25 M, 0.5 N. Dissolve 74 gm of $Zn(NO_3)_2.6H_2O$ in 1 liter of water.

Zinc sulfate, 0.25 M, 0.5 N. Dissolve 72 gm of $ZnSO_4.7H_2O$ in 1 liter of water.

Special Solutions and Reagents

Aluminon *(qualitative test for aluminum)*. Aluminon is a trade name for the ammonium salt of aurin tricarboxylic acid. Dissolve 1 gm of the salt in 1 liter of distilled water. Shake the solution well to insure thorough mixing.

Ammonia-Ammonium Chloride Solution Strong(Ammonia buffer), Dissolve ammonium chloride (67.5 gm) in strong ammonia solution (740 ml) and add sufficient water to produce 1000 ml.

Ammonium Acetate Solution, Dissolve ammonium acetate (150 gm) in water (200 ml). Add glacial acetic acid (3 ml) and dilute to 1000 ml with water.

Anisaldehyde-Acetic Acid Reagent, Mix Anisaldehyde (0.5 ml) with 98% acetic acid (10 ml).

Anisaldehyde-Sulphuric Acid Reagent, Mix Anisaldehyde (0.5 ml) with glacial acetic acid (10 ml), followed by addition of methanol (85 ml) and concentrated sulphuric acid (5 ml).

Bang's reagent *(for glucose estimation)*. Dissolve 100 gm of K_2CO_3, 66 gm of KCl and 160 of $KHCO_3$ in the order given in about 700 ml of water at 30°C. Add 4.4 gm of $CuSO_4$ and dilute to 1 liter after the CO_2 is evolved. This solution should be shaken only in such a manner as not to allow entry of air. After 24 hours 300 ml are diluted to 1 liter with saturated KCl solution, shaken gently and used after 24 hours; 50 ml equivalent to 10 mg glucose.

Barfoed's reagent *(test for glucose).* See Cupric acetate.

Baudisch's reagent. *See Cupferron.*

Benedict's solution *(qualitative reagent for glucose).* With the aid of heat, dissolve 173 gm of sodium citrate and 100 gm of Na_2CO_3 in 800 ml of water. Filter, if necessary, and dilute to 850 ml. Dissolve 17.3 gm of $CuSO_4.5H_2O$ in 100 ml of water. Pour the latter solution, with constant stirring, into the carbonate-citrate solution, and make up to 1 liter.

Benzidine hydrochloride solution *(for sulphate determination).* Make a paste of 8 gm of benzidine hydrochloride $(C_{12}H_8(NH_2)_2.2HCl)$ and 20 ml of water, add 20 ml of HCl (sp. gr. 1.12) and dilute to 1 liter with water. Each ml of this solution is equivalent to 0.00357 gm of H_2SO_4.

Bertrand's reagent *(glucose estimation).* Consists of the following solutions:

(a) Dissolve 200g of Rochelle salts and 150 gm of NaOH in sufficient water to make 1 liter of solution.

(b) Dissolve 40 gm of CuSO4 in enough water to make 1 liter of solution.

(c) Dissolve 50 gm of $Fe_2(SO_4)_3$ and 200g of H_2SO_4 (sp. gr. 1.84) in sufficient water to make 1 liter of solution.

(d) Dissolve 5 gm of KMnO4 in sufficient water to make 1 liter of solution.

Blal's reagent *(for pentose).* Dissolve 1g of orcinol $(CH_3.C_6H_3(OH)_2)$ in 500 ml of 30% HCl to which 30 drops of a 10% solution of $FeCl_3$ has been added.

Brucke's reagent *(protein precipitation).* See Potassium iodide-mercuric iodide.

Bromine Solution, Dissolve bromine (9.6 ml) and potassium bromide (30 gm) in sufficient water to produce 100 ml.

Bromine Water : Saturate water with bromine by shaking about 10 ml of bromine in one litre of water.

Ceric Ammonium Sulphate, Suspend Ceric sulphate (1 gm) in water (40 ml). Add trichloroacetic acid (10 gm), slowly add drop by drop sulphuric acid (d 1.84), until the solution clarifies.

Chlorinated Lime Solution : Mix chlorinated lime (100.gm) with water (1000 ml), transfer the mixture to a stoppered bottle, set aside for three hours, shaking occasionally and filter through calico. Chlorinated lime must be prepared freshly.

Cobalticyanide paper *(Rinnmann's test for Zn).* Dissolve 4 gm of $K_2Co(CN)_5$ and 1g of $KClO_3$ in 100 ml of water. Soak filter paper in solution and dry at 100° C. Apply drop of zinc solution and burn in an evaporating dish. A green disk is obtained if zinc is present.

Cochineal. Extract 1 gm of cochineal for four days with 20 ml of alcohol and 60 ml of distilled water. Filter.

Congo red. Dissolve 0.5 gm of congo red in 90 ml of distilled water and 10 ml of alcohol.

Cupferron *(Baudisch 's reagent for iron analysis).* Dissolve 6 gm of the ammonium salt of nitroso-phenyl-hydroxyl-amine (cupferron) in 100 ml of H_2O. Reagent good for one week only and must be kept in the dark.

Cupric acetate (*Barfoed's reagent for reducing monosaccharides*), dissolve 66 gm of cupric acetate and 10 ml of glacial acetic acid in water and dilute to 1 liter.

Cupric oxide, ammoniacal (*Schweitzer's reagent*), (dissolves cotton, linen and silk, but not wool):

1. Dissolve 5 gm of cupric sulfate in 100 ml of boiling water, and add sodium hydroxide until precipitation is complete. Wash the precipitate well, and dissolve it in a minimum quantity of ammonium hydroxide.

2. Bubble a slow stream of air through 300 ml of strong ammonium hydroxide containing 50g of fine copper turnings. Continue for one hour.

Cupric sulphate in glycerin-potassium hydroxide (*reagent for silk*), dissolve 10 gm of cupric sulphate, $CuSO_4.5H_2O$, in 100 ml of water and add 5 gm of glycerin. Add KOH solution slowly until a deep blue solution is obtained.

Cupron (*benzoin oxime*). Dissolve 5 gm in 100 ml of 95 % alcohol.

Cuprous chloride, acidic (*reagent for CO in gas analysis*),

1. Cover the bottom of a two-liter flask with a layer of cupric oxide about one-half inch deep, suspend a bunch of copper wire so as to reach from the bottom to the top of the solution, and fill the flask with hydrochloric acid (sp. gr. 1.10). Shake occasionally. When the solution becomes nearly colorless, transfer to reagent bottles, which should also contain copper wire. The stock bottle may be refilled with dilute hydrochloric acid until either the cupric oxide or the copper wire is used up.

   Copper sulfate may be substituted for copper oxide in the above procedure.

2. Dissolve 340 gm of $CuCl_2.2H_2O$ in 600 ml of conc. HCl and reduce the cupric chloride by adding 190 ml of a saturated solution of stannous chloride or until the solution is colorless. The stannous chloride is prepared by treating 300 gm of metallic tin in a 500 ml flask with conc. HCl until no more tin goes into solution.

3. *Winkler method* : Add a mixture of 86 gm of CuO and 17 gm of finely divided metallic Cu, made by the reduction of CuO with hydrogen, to a solution of HCl, made by diluting 650 ml of conc. HCl with 325 ml of water. After the mixture has been added slowly and with frequent stirring, a spiral of copper wire is suspended in the bottle, reaching all the way to the bottom. Shake occasionally, and when the solution becomes colorless, it is ready for use.

Cuprous chloride, ammoniacal (*reagent for CO in gas analysis*),

1. The acid solution of cuprous chloride as prepared above is neutralized with ammonium hydroxide until an ammonia odor persists. An excess of metallic copper must be kept in the solution.

2. Pour 800 ml of acidic cuprous chloride, prepared by the Winkler method, into about 4 liters of water. Transfer the precipitate to a 250 ml graduate. After several hours, siphon off the liquid above the 50 ml mark and refill with 7.5% NH_4OH solution which may be prepared by diluting 50 ml of conc. NH_4OH with 150 ml of water. The solution is well shaken and allowed to stand for several hours. It should have a faint odor of ammonia.

2, 6-Dichlorophenolindophenol Solution, Warm 2, 6-dichlorophenolindophenol sodium salt (0.1 gm) with water (100 ml) and filter.

Dichlorfluorescin indicator, Dissolve 1 gm in 1 liter of 70% alcohol or 1 gm of the sodium salt in 1 liter of water.

Dimethylglyoxime (diacetyl dioxime), 0.01 N. Dissolve 0.6 gm of dimethylglyoxime, $(CH_3CNOH)_2$, in 500 ml of 95 % ethyl alcohol. This is an especially sensitive test for nickel, a very definite crimson color being produced.

2, 4-Dinitrophenylhydrazine, Dissolve 2, 4-dinitrophenylhydrazine (2 gm) in concentrated sulphuric acid (10 ml). Add sufficient ethanol to produce 200 ml.

Diphenylamine *(reagent for rayon),* Dissolve 0.2 gm in 100 ml of concentrated sulfuric acid.

Diphenylamine sulfonate *(for titration of iron with $K_2Cr_2O_7$),* Dissolve 0.32 gm of the barium salt of diphenylamine sulfonic acid in 100 ml of water, add 0.5 gm of sodium sulphate and filter off the precipitate of BaSO4.

Diphenylcarbazide, Dissolve 0.2 gm of diphenylcarbazide in 10 ml of glacial acetic acid and dilute to 100 ml with 95% ethyl alcohol.

Dragendorff's Reagent, (A) Boil bismuth carbonate (2.6 gm) and sodium iodide (7.0 gm) for few minute with glacial acetic acid (25 ml). After 12 hrs, filter off the precipitated sodium acetate crystals. To the 20 ml of the clear red-brown filtrate, mix the ethyl acetate (8 ml) and store in a brown bottle. (B) Dissolve basic bismuth nitrate (0.85 gm) in water (40 ml) and glacial acetic acid (10 ml) followed by addition of potassium iodide (8 gm) dissolved in water (20 ml).

Esbach's reagent *(estimation of protein),* To a water solution of 10 gm of picric acid and 20g of citric acid, add sufficient water to make one liter of solution.

Fehling's solution, *(reagent for reducing sugars):*

Fehling Solution A, Dissolve crystalline copper sulphate (34.64 gm) in water (500 ml) containing a few drops of concentrated sulphuric acid.

Fehling Solution B, Dissolve sodium potassium tartrate (Rochelle salt) (173 gm) and sodium hydroxide (60 gm) in water and make the solution to 500 ml with water.

For use, mix equal volumes of the two solutions at the time of using.

Ferric-alum indicator, Dissolve 140 gm of ferric-ammonium sulfate crystals in 400 ml of hot water. When cool, filter, and make up to a volume of 500 ml with dilute (6 N) nitric acid.

Folin's mixture, *(for uric acid),* To 650 ml of water add 500 gm of (NH4)2SO4, 5 gm of uranium acetate and 6 gm of glacial acetic acid. Dilute to 1 liter.

Formaldehyde-sulphuric acid *(Marquis' reagent for alkaloids),* Add 10 ml of formaldehyde solution to 50 ml of sulphuric acid.

Froehde's reagent, See Sulphomolybdic actid.

Fuchsin *(reagent for linen).* Dissolve 1g of fuchsin in 100 ml of alcohol.

Fuchsin-sulphurous acid *(Schiff's reagent for aldehydes),* Dissolve 0.5 gm of fuchsin and 9 gm of sodium bisulfite in 500 ml of water, and add 10 ml of HCI. Keep in well-stoppered bottles and protect from light.

Gunzberg's reagent *(detection of HCl in gastric juice)*, Prepare as needed a solution containing 4 gm of phloroglucinol and 2 gm of vanillin in 100 ml of absolute ethyl alcohol.

Hager's reagent, See Picric acid.

To 50 ml of water add 70 gm of I2 and 50 gm of KI. Dilute to 1 liter with alcohol.

Iodo-potasium iodide *(Wagner's reagent for alkaloids)*, Dissolve 2 gm of iodine and 6 gm of KI in 100 ml of water.

Kedde Reagent, Mix freshly prepared ethanolic 3, 5-dinitrobenzoic acid solution (5 ml) with 2M sodium hydroxide solution (5 ml).

Lead Acetate Solution, A 10% w/v solution of lead acetate in carbon dioxide free water.

Liebermann-Burchard Reagent, Add acetic anhydride (5 ml) and concentrated sulphuric acid (5 ml) carefully to absolute ethanol (5 ml), while cooling in ice. The reagent must be freshly prepared.

Litmus (indicator), Extract litmus powder three times with boiling alcohol, each treatment consuming an hour. Reject the alcoholic extract. Treat residue with an equal weight of cold water and. filter; then exhaust with five times its weight of boiling water, cool and filter. Combine the aqueous extracts.

Magnesia mixture *(reagent for phosphates and arsenates)*, Dissolve 55 gm of magnesium chloride and 105 gm of ammonium chloride in water, barely acidify with hydrochloric acid, and dilute to 1 liter. The ammonium hydroxide may be omitted until just previous to use. The reagent, if completely mixed and stored for any period of time, becomes turbid.

Magnesium uranyl acetate, Dissolve 100 gm of $UO_2(C_2H_3O_2)_2.2H_2O$ in 60 ml of glacial acetic acid and dilute to 500 ml. Dissolve 330 gm of $mg(C_2H_3O_2)_2.4H_2O$ in 60 ml of glacial acetic acid and dilute to 200 ml. Heat solutions to the boiling point until clear, pour the magnesium solution into time uranyl solution, cool and dilute to 1 liter. Let stand over night and filter if necessary.

Marme's reagent, See Potassium-cadmium iodide.

Marqui's reagent, See Formaldehyde-sulfuric acid.

Mayer's reagent, *(white precipitate with most alkaloids in slightly acid solutions)*. Dissolve 1.358 gm of $HgCl_2$ in 60 ml of water and pour into a solution of 5 gm of KI in 10 ml of H2O Add sufficient water to make 100 ml.

Methyl orange indicator, Dissolve 1 gm of methyl orange in 1 liter of water. Filter, if necessary.

Methyl orange, modified, Dissolve 2 gm of methyl orange and 2.8 gm of xylene cyanole in 1 liter of 50% alcohol.

Methyl red indicator, Dissolve 1 gm of methyl red in 600 ml of alcohol and dilute with 400 ml of water.

Methyl red, modified, Dissolve 0.50 gmof methyl red and 1.25 gm of xylene cyanole in 1 liter of 90% alcohol. Or, dissolve 1.25 gm of methyl red and 0.825 gm of methylene blue in 1 liter of 90% alcohol.

Millon's reagent *(for albumins and phenols),* Dissolve 1 part of mercury in 1 part of cold fuming nitric acid. Dilute with twice the volume of water and decant the clear solution after several hours.

Mixed indicator, Prepared by adding about 1.4 gm of xyleno cyanole FF to 1 gm of methyl orange. The dye Is seldom pure enough for these proportion to be satisfactory. Each new lot of dye should be tested by adding additional amounts of the dye until test portion gives the proper color change. The acid color of this indicator Is like that of permanganate; the neutral color is gray; and the alkaline color Is green. Described by Hickman and Linstead, J. Chem. Soc. (Lon.), 121, 2502 (1922).

Molisch's reagent, See a-Naphthol.

α-**Naphthol** *(Molisch's reagent for wool),* Dissolve 15 gm of a-naphthol in 100 ml of alcohol or chloroform.

Nessler's reagent *(for ammoniak),* Dissolve 50 gm of KI in the smallest possible quantity of cold water (50 ml). Add a saturated solution of mercuric chloride (about 22 gm in 350 ml of water will be needed) until an excess is indicated by the formation of a precipitate. Then add 200 ml of 5N NaOH and dilute to 1 liter. Let settle, and draw off the clear liquid.

Ninhydrin Reagent, Dissolve ninhydrin (30 mg) in n-butanol (10 ml), followed by 98% of acetic acid (0.3 ml).

Nitron *(detection of nitrate radical),* Dissolve 10 gm of nitron ($C_{20}H_{16}N_4$, 4,5-dihydro-1,4-diphenyl-3,5-phenylimino-1,2,4-triazole) in 5 ml of glacial acetic acid and 95 ml of water. The solution may be filtered with slight suction through an alundum crucible and kept in a dark bottle.

Nylander's solution (carbohydrates), Dissolve 20 gm of bismuth subnitrate and 40 gm of Rochelle salts in 1 liter of 8% NaOH solution. Cool and filter.

Oxine. Dissolve 14 m of HC_9H_6ON in 30 ml of glacial acetic acid. Warm slightly, if necessary. Dilute to 1 liter.

Pasteur's salt solution, To one liter of distilled water add 2.5 gm of potassium phosphate, 0.25 gm of calcium phosphates, 0.25 gm of magnesium sulfate and 12.00g of ammonium tartrate.

Pavy's solution *(glucose reagent),* To 120 ml of Fehling's solution, add 300 ml of NH_4OH (sp. gr. 0.88) and dilute to 1 liter with water.

Phenanthroline ferrous ion indicator, Dissolve 1.485 gm of phenanthroline monohydrate in 100 ml of 0.025 M ferrous sulfate solution.

Phenolphthalein, Dissolve 1 gm of phenolphthalein in 50 ml of alcohol and add 50 ml of water.

Phenylhydrazine Solution, Dissolve phenylhydrazine hydrochloride (65 gm) previously recrystallizedfrom aqueous ethanol in sufficient mixture of sulphuric acid (70 ml) and water (30 ml) to produce 100 ml.

Phloroglucinol solution *(pentosans),* Make a 3% phloroglucinol solution in alcohol. Keep in a dark bottle.

Phosphomolybdic acid *(Sonnenschein 's reagent for alkaloids)*:

1. Prepare ammonium phosphomolybdate and after washing with water, boil with nitric acid and expel NH_3; evaporate to dryness and dissolve in 2 N nitric acid.

2. Dissolve ammonium molybdate in HNO_3, and treat with phosphoric acid. Filter, wash the precipitate, and boil with aqua regia until the ammonium salt is decomposed. Evaporate to dryness. The residue dissolved in 10% HNO_3 constitutes Sonnenschein's reagent.

Phosphoric acid - sulphuric acid mixture, Dilute 150 ml of conc. H_2SO_4 and 100 ml of conc. H_3PO_4 (85%) with water to a volume of 1 liter.

Phosphotungstic acid *(Scheibler 's reagent for alkaloids)*,

1. Dissolve 20 gm of sodium tungstate and 15 g of sodium phosphate in 100 ml of water containing a little nitric acid.

2. The reagent is a 10% solution of phosphotungstic acid in water. The phosphotungstic acid is prepared by evaporating a mixture of 10g of sodium tungstate dissolved in 5 g of phosphoric acid (sp. gr. 1.13) and enough boiling water to effect solution. Crystals of phosphotungstic acid separate.

Picric acid *(Hager 's reagent for alkaloids, wool and silk)*, Dissolve 1 gm of picric acid in 100 ml of water.

Potassium antimonate *(reagent for sodium)*, Boil 22 gm of potassium antimonate with 1 liter of water until nearly all of the salt has dissolved, cool quickly, and add 35 ml of 10% potassium hydroxide. Filter after standing over night.

Potassium hydroxide *(for CO_2 absorption)*, Dissolve 360 gm of KOH in water and dilute to 1 liter.

Potassium iodide-mercuric iodide *(Brucke's reagent for proteins)*, Dissolve 50 gm of KI in 500 ml of water, and saturate with mercuric iodide (about 120 g). Dilute to 1 liter.

Potassium pyrogallate *(for oxygen absorption)*, For mixtures of gases containing less than 28% oxygen, add 100 ml of KOH solution (50 g of KOH to 100 ml of water) to 5g of pyrogallol. For mixtures containing more than 28% oxygen the KOH solution should contain 120 gm of KOH to 100 ml of water.

Potassium-cadmium iodide *(Marme's reagent for alkaloids)*, Add 2 gm of CdI2 to a boiling solution of 4 gm of KI in 12 ml of water, and then mix with 12 ml of saturated KI solution.

Potassium Mercuri-iodide Solution (Mayer's Reagent), Add aqueous mercuric chloride (1.36 gm in 60 ml of water) solution to a solution of potassium iodide (5 gm) in water (20 ml), mix and add sufficient water to produce 100 ml.

Potassium Mercuri-iodide Solution, (Alkaline Nessler Reagent), To potassium iodide (3.5 gm), add mercuric chloride (1.25 gm) dissolved in water (80 ml), add cold saturated solution of mercuric chloride in water with constant stirring until a slight red precipitate remains. Dissolve sodium hydroxide (12 gm) in the solution, add a little more of the cold saturated solution of mercuric chloride and sufficient water to produce 100 ml. Allow to stand and **decant** the clear liquid.

Potassium Permanganate Solution (Baeyer's Reagent), Dissolve potassium permanganate (1 gm) in water (100 ml) and add few drops of potassium hydroxide solution to it to get clear pink colour solution.

Pyridine Bromide Solution : Dissolve pyridine (10 ml) and sulphuric acid (5.4 ml) in glacial acetic acid (20 ml) keeping the mixture cool. Add bromine (2.6 ml) dissolved in glacial acetic acid (20 ml) and dilute with glacial acetic acid to 100 ml.Pyridine bromide solution should be freshly prepared.

Pyrogallol, alkaline,

(a) Dissolve 75 gm of pyrogallic acid in 75 ml of water.

(b) Dissolve 500 gm of KOH in 250 ml of water. When cool, adjust until sp. gr. is 1.55.

For use, add 270 ml of solution (b) to 30 ml of solution (a).

Scheibler's reagent, See Phosphotungstic acid.

Schiff's reagent, See Fuchsin-sulphurous acid.

Sodium hydroxide *(for CO2 absorption)*, Dissolve 330 gm of NaOH in water and dilute to 1 liter.

Sodium nitroprusside *(reagent for hydrogen sulphide and wool)*, Use a freshly prepared solution of 1 gm of sodium nitroprusside in 10 ml of water.

Sodium oxalate, Dissolve 30 gm of the commercial salt in 1 liter of water, make slightly alkaline with sodium hydroxide, and let stand until perfectly clear. Filter and evaporate the filtrate to 100 ml. Cool and filter. Pulverize the residue and wash it several times with small volumes of water. The procedure is repeated until the mother liquor is free from sulfate and is neutral to phenolphthalein.

Sodium plumbite *(reagent for wool)*, Dissolve 5 gm of sodium hydroxide in 100 ml of water. Add 5 gm of litharge and boil until dissolved.

Sodium polysulphide, Dissolve 480 gm of $Na_2S.9H_2O$ in 500 ml of water, add 40 gm of NaOH and 18 gm of sulfur. Stir thoroughly and dilute to 1 liter with water.

Sonnenschein's reagent, See Phosphomolybdic acid.

Starch solution,

1. Make a paste with 2 gm of soluble starch and 0.01 gm of HgI_2 with a small amount of water. Add the mixture slowly to 1 liter of boiling water and boil for a few minutes. Keep in a glass stoppered bottle. If other than soluble starch is used, the solution will not clear on boiling; it should be allowed to stand and the clear liquid decanted.

2. A solution of starch which keeps indefinitely is made as follows: Mix 500 ml of saturated NaCl solution (filtered), 80 ml of glacial acetic acid, 20 ml of water and 3 gm of starch. Bring slowly to a boil and boil for two minutes.

3. Make a paste with 1 gm of soluble starch and 5 mg of HgI_2, using as little cold water as possible. Then pour about 200 ml of boiling water on the paste and stir immediately. This will give a clear solution if the paste is prepared correctly and the water actually boiling. Cool

and add 4g of KI. Starch solution decomposes on standing due to bacterial action, but this solution will keep a long time if stored under a layer of toluene.

Stoke's reagent, Dissolve 30 gm of $FeSO_4$ and 20 gm of tartaric acid in water and dilute to 1 liter. Just before using, add concentrated NH_4OH until the precipitate first formed is redissolved.

Tannic acid *(reagent for albumen, alkaloids and gelatin)*, Dissolve 10 gm of tannic acid in 10 ml of alcohol and dilute with water to 100 ml.

Trinitrophenol solution, See Picric acid.

Tannic Acid Solution, A 10% w/v solution of tannic acid in water (100 ml).

Thioacetamide Reagent, Add 1 ml of a mixture of N sodium hydroxide (15 ml), water (5 ml) and glycerin (20 ml) to a 4% w/v solution of thioacetamide (0.2 ml) in water. Heat on water bath for twenty seconds and cool.Thioacetamide reagent should be prepared immediately before use.

o-Tolidine solution (residual chlorine in water analysis), Prepare 1 liter of dilute HCl (100 ml of HCl (sp. gr. 1.19) in sufficient water to make 1 liter). Dissolve 1 gm of o-tolidine in 100 ml of the dilute HCl and dilute to 1 liter with dilute HCl solution.

Trinitrophenol solution, See Picric acid.

Uffelmann's reagent *(turns yellow in presence of a lactic acid)*, To a 2% solution of pure phenol in water, add a water solution of FeCl3 until the phenol solution hecornes violet in color.

Vanillin-Hydrochloric Acid Reagent, Dissolve Vanillin (1 gm) in ethanol (100 ml) and then add concentrated hydrochloric acid (3 ml) to it.

Vanillin-Sulphuric Acid Reagent, Dissolve Vanillin (1 gm) in ethanol (100 ml) and then add concentrated sulphuric acid (3 ml) to it.

Wagner's reagent, See Iodo-potassium iodide.

Wagner's solution (used in phosphate rock analysis to prevent precipitation of iron and aluminum), Dissolve 25g of citric acid and 1g of salicylic acid in water and dilute to 1 liter. Use 50 ml of the reagent.

Wij's iodine monochloride solution *(for iodine number)*, Dissolve 13 gm of resublimed iodine in 1 liter of glacial acetic acid which will pass the dichromate test for reducible matter. Set aside 25 ml of this solution. Pass into the remainder of the solution dry chlorine gas (dried and washed by passing through H_2SO_4 (sp. Gr. 1.84)) until the characteristic color of free iodine has been discharged. Now add the iodine solution which was reserved, until all free chlorine has been destroyed. A slight excess of iodine does little or no harm, but an excess of chlorine must be avoided. Preserve in well stoppered, amber colored bottles. Avoid use of solutions which have been prepared for more than 30 days.

Wij's special solution (for iodine number-Analyst 58, 523-7, 1933), To 200 ml of glacial acetic acid that will pass the dichromate test for reducible matter, add 12g of dichloroamine T (paratoluene-sulfonedichloroamide), and 16.6 gm of dry KI (in small quantities with continual shaking until all the

KI has dissolved). Make up to 1 liter with the same quality of acetic acid used above and preserve in a dark colored bottle.

Zimmermann-Reinhardt reagent (determination of iron), Dissolve 70g of $MnSO_4.4H_2O$ in 500 ml of water, add 125 ml of oonc.H_2SO_4 and 125 ml of 85% H_3PO_4, and dilute to 1 liter.

Zinc chloride solution, basic *(reagent for silk)*, Dissolve 1000 gm of zinc chloride in 850 ml of water, and add 40g of zinc oxide. Heat until solution is complete.

Zinc uranyl acetate *(reagent for sodium)*, Dissolve 10 gm of $UO_2(C_2H_3O_2)_2.2H_2O$ in 6 gm of 30 % acetic acid with heat, if necessary, and dilute to 50 ml. Dissolve 30 gm of $Zn(C_2H_3O_2)_2.2H_2O$ in 3g of 30% acetic acid and dilute to 50 ml. Mix the two solutions, add 50 mg of NaCl, allow to stand over night and filter.

Index